This is dedicated to and in memory of our wife, mother, grandmother, sister, daughter, and friend Tina. You are the reason for who we all are today. We all miss you more than words can express. Please watch over us and our children. Fly high, we love you!

I0464191

She never woke up this morning
She will never take another breath
She will never shed another tear
She is no longer in pain
She is home
She is whole again in spirit
She is whole again in peace
Her smile will live on forever
In every memory that she made
She showed love, mercy, strength,
Compassion, forgiveness, truth and trust
Heavenly Father bless this woman as you
Have welcomed her into your gates
Rest in peace sweet lady,
I love you Tina.
Written by Amanda H.

Amy R., Coworker- *"So glad she was a part of my life and I was a part of hers."*

Debbie M., Family friend- *"She was a wonderful person inside and out. I miss her and love her. I thank her for my wonderful memories."*

Robyn S., Friend, Cancer survivor- *"I was just thinking about her earlier and how sometimes I still want to just call her. I just have to snap out of it. I sure miss her."*

Ashley H., Daughter- *"My mom did not have much of a sense of humor. My favorite memory of her is from one of the few times a little tiny bit of humor showed its face.*

Mom- *""What's wrong?""*

Me- *""My arm itches.""*

Mom- *""I think there is some jerking lotion in there.""*

Me- *""Uhm jerking? No thanks mom!!""*

Mom- (laughing hysterically)*""Jergens, I meant Jergens! But it is your brother's so...."*

Me- *""Yea, uhm no thanks!""*

We laughed until we were both crying. Mom was not normally like this so it was nice to have a good laugh with her."

Debbie D., Family friend- *"One of my first memories is soon after we moved in our house, your mom and I became quick friends. It was April fool's Day; I called your mom and told her someone was on the roof of her house. Now mind you, we only lived in our house a couple weeks and I did that. She came running outside in her pajamas, running through the yard trying to see who was up there while I was in the house laughing my ass off. I don't think she was mad. I did the same thing the next year, but she didn't fall for it that time. I miss that friend."*

Carla L., Family friend- *"I remember the first time my family met your family. I believe you and Heather were in the 3rd grade. It was my first paid vacation I had ever had. I know about half way from Oklahoma to Illinois I started to worry if our families would like each other. As soon as Tina and I met it was like we had known each other a long time. Over the years we wrote letters, called each other when we were happy, sad or very mad!!!!! Oh how I miss those talks!!!"*

"I remember the day Tina called me and told me she had cancer. Even then she was telling me it would be okay. I totally lost it after that phone call. My friend tried to comfort me and tell me that it would be okay. The next day I worked I told my boss I had to go see her. I was prepared to lose my job if I had to!!! I was nervous because I had never gone out of state by myself. Plus my arthritis had been bad so I wasn't sure if I could make the trip. That trip ended up being good for me as well as Tina. I got her up off the couch and she made me walk. She told her family she had quit smoking but she hadn't. She had cut back; I knew her hiding place for her cigarettes."

Brianna T., Granddaughter- *'My favorite memory of grandma was when she had you all fooled that she had stopped smoking. She would sneak out side to the neighbor's house where had a bunch of stuff stacked out there and hide and smoke while her and I talked, she told me never to tell anyone and I didn't"*

Tammy C., Sister-*"I remember the day we found out my sister had cancer. She was in the hospital in isolation because they didn't know what she had until they did the biopsy. The doctors came into the room and said I am sorry to say but you have lung cancer. My heart just about quit right then. This was the day before my birthday June 15, 2012. I started crying and Tina looked at me and said it's going to be okay, I am going to fight this. I have to see and raise my grandbabies, I am going to fight this, don't cry sis it's going to be okay. Me and her were born 11 months and 12 days apart. We shared a room together growing up. We were best friends. We called each other at least once a week to talk. She put up a hell of a fight. I came over and stayed on a Friday night so Bryon and Ashley could get a good night's sleep right before she passed and I was taking her to the bathroom and she looked down at my shoes and said those are the ugliest damn shoes I have ever seen sis. All I could do was laugh. I miss her more and more every day. R.I.P. sis I love you to the moon and back!"*

Rayleigh G., Granddaughter- *"My favoritest memory of grandma was when she let me do her make-up outside with chalk."*

Kristina D., Family friend- *"I remember the night she found out I was pregnant with Alyssa!!!! We pulled up to your house to tell your mom you were staying with me at like 10pm and she said no. And your response to her was YES I AM. You had to end up telling her, we had to drive to Lake Fork to tell Nick I was pregnant. That next morning when I dropped you off at your house mama bear came out and told me "" Honey, I know what's going on and you have to tell your mom."" instantly tears start going down my cheek and she promised me everything would be ok. After Alyssa was born she gave me a blanket she had made!!!!!!!"*

Amy P., Family friend- *"My fondest memory of your mom was the love and pride she had for her family and friends. She had unconditional love for us all. She beamed with pride on her children's accomplishments as well as her friend's children. The smile on her face as she took a picture (we all know she took a picture or two) is something I will never forget."*

Doug W., Family friend-*"I remember when your mom was taking pictures our senior year. I told her no pictures. She said Doug stop bitching. It's your last first day of school. When I worked at the gas station and I was having a bad day she could make it better. Her face when I asked for her ID was priceless."*

Dylan H., Grandson- *"I remember grandma wanted me to hug her and I wouldn't and started to laugh."*

Missy H., Sister- *"Ask your Dad about it but I believe he said with our drastic age difference of 16 years she apparently used me as a way to go on a date with your Father!! I know she also used to take me to the mall all the time with the other Sisters to shop and they got my ears pierced when I was like 2 or 3 there as well!! And one time she came into the bar that Dad was at (not really sure which one) and I was laying there sleeping on the bar as an infant!! Your Mother got so mad at Dad and she picked me up and took me out of there as fast as she could!! Plus when I got pregnant I planned to tell everyone together at Dad's 74th birthday party at Salisbury Bar!! So I go up to tell your Mom and say sis I have something to tell you!! I'm pregnant and all she has to say is I know!! I said really and she says yes!! She always had a way of knowing things!! Also the whole time I was pregnant she told me I was having a boy and she has never been wrong she said!! When referring to the baby she would say my Nephew so of course when I told her I was having a girl she was like no way!! She said of course coming from you!! You had to break my streak didn't you!! She also was so upset because her surgery was set and they were going put those radioactive beads in her and when I had the baby (due December 26th) or still while I was pregnant I wasn't going able to come around while she had those in her!! Then she called me super excited and said that they didn't see a reason to put so many in her and that she would be able to see the Olivea shortly after I had her!!"*

Bradley T., Grandson- *" I used to spit a lot and I remember grandma put a rubber band around my wrist and every time she caught me spitting she would snap the rubber band."*

Destiny H., Granddaughter- *"I remember grandma always used to let me paint her nails when I came to visit."*

"One of the last times grandma and grandpa came to visit they brought Rayleigh up with them. Rayleigh and I were dancing around the living room. Grandma got up with her cane and started to dance with me and Rayleigh. That is my favorite memory of grandma"

Damon H., Son- *"My favorite memory of mom was when Jamie and I were shooting rubber bands at each other and I accidentally hit her. She said she would get me back when I least expected it. Later on that day she caught me in the kitchen, body* slammed me and held the rubber band to my skin and laughed saying ""You'll never hit me again will you?"' It was hilarious."

Amanda H., Daughter-in-law- *"Tina was the mother-in-law that every girl dreams of and for a short time I got to have her."*

Kortni B., Family friend- *"Your mom was the best librarian ever! I remember she used to read to me and my little sisters all the time."*

Roberta L., Family friend- *"Your mom was and still is a wonderful person and she had a great heart. I remember when I first moved to Illiopolis. I had put the kids to bed and went to peel an orange and cut the damn top of my thumb off. I had one of the girls go get her and she helped me, it was bleeding badly. Your mother always was a very happy person. She was always smiling, loved her flower and working in the yard. She loved loved loved Reba."*

Prologue

Each and every person will face death at some point in their life whether it is tragic and unexpected or a terminal illness that is expected. No matter which way it happens it is not easy to deal with, especially if it is someone you are very close to such as a child, parent, sibling or spouse. I hear all the time "Well at least you got to say goodbye." Or "Be glad it was sudden and they did not have to suffer." Is there really a right or wrong way to die? Is one way better than the other? These are questions I have always wondered the answer to, especially these past few months. You either suffer, struggle or lie in bed wondering will today be the day? Will I make it until supper time tonight? Will my family be okay without me here? Or you are taken suddenly leaving your family shocked, surprised and scrambling to figure out how they will manage expenses and life without you there. It is funny how you never realize the impact of someone's presences until they are no longer there, you cannot just drop in to say hello or pick up the phone and call them. Your daily habits are thrown way out of whack and you have to completely adjust your life to suit their absence. My point here is no matter whether it is sudden or to be expected you still have to do a lot of adjusting. You may feel as if your life is over, having no reasons left to live yourself. I felt this way myself a time or two, but I look at my daughter and realize I have a lot left to live for. If you are to gain one thing from this story I want it to be that life doesn't have to be over, you do not have to spiral downwards into an emotional mess or do the unthinkable and commit suicide. Even though it may feel as if life is over, please take a step back and think how you felt when you lost the special someone, the pain, tears and heartbreak. You too are that special someone to another person, can you really put them through what you yourself just experienced? Death is tragic, no one can deny this. Please realize you can live on in their memories. You are strong enough to dust off and continue on. We do not ever have to forget about our loved ones who we have lost. They are with us, only in a different way and it is our job to share those memories with the younger generations who may not have had the pleasure of meeting our lost loved ones. It is our responsibility to keep their spirits alive; we cannot do this if we ourselves choose not to live on. Help them fly high!

It was like any other cold and dreary day in March. For me it was a little extra special. It was my birthday week and my mom Tina and my youngest brother Damon were driving three hours to come visit with my daughter Rayleigh and I. Little did we all know that weekend would be the start of a hellacious two year journey, ending in a life changing, traumatic event for my whole entire family.

Tina was a very kind hearted person, who befriended every person she met and was very likable. She cherished each and every friend she had, no matter how long they had known each other. That woman didn't have a mean bone in her body. Someone could say something mean about her and my mom still treated them as if they were one of her lifelong friends. Tina never defended herself to anyone, she preferred to let people talk and turn the other cheek. I have never met anyone who cared so much about their family and was always the middle man trying to make things right between whoever was fighting at the moment. I remember a time my brother Damon and I got into a fist fight; we were determined to kill each other. My mother jumped right in the middle of flying hands and feet to try to keep the peace. You always hear the saying "He would give you the shirt off his back." Well she really would give you the shirt off her back, no questions asked, and expected nothing in return. My mom was very active in our lives growing up all seven of us, yes you read that right seven children Bryon, Jason, Nathan, Danny, myself, Jamie and Damon. The four older boys, Bryon, Jason, Nathan and Danny were my dad's from previous marriages but you dare not call them stepchildren. They were her son's and Tina was proud to have them in her life. Not one of us kids, biological or not were treated any different than the next. The punishments were the same across the board. I recall a time mom asked Nathan and I to clean our bedrooms. We thought it would be a great idea to shove everything in the closet and under the beds. Mom was stupid right? We never thought she would look under the bed or check the closets? Nathan lost his car and I lost my bicycle for two weeks, not to mention we had to re-clean the entire room and to mom's standards. She made it to every single game, event or concert we had sick or not my mom was there, camera in hand, smile on her face and there were a lot of them through the years. When all of us kids started to have kids of our own the excitement really set in, she loved her grand babies more than life itself. There are twelve grandkids total. Bryon has three boys Bryce, Krue, and Rylan. Jason has a boy named Nolan and a little girl named Alexis, but we all call her Lexi. Nathan has four children two boys and two girls Bradley, Brianna, Destiny and Dylan. I have one child her name is Rayleigh. Jamie has a little boy named Noah. Damon has a little girl named Jaycee. If any of us kids were dating someone who had children, they were hers as well. No one ever gets left out or treated like an outcast around my mom. There were presents, birthday parties, hugs and kisses for every single one of the grandkids, blood or not. We could show up to the house, drop the kids off for a month and leave, mom wouldn't care one single bit. She always told us "Don't you dare come over without my babies." Tina meant it! Scrap booking was one of her favorite things to do. I still look at the scrapbooks she made for Rayleigh and me. Her intentions were to make one for each of us kids from birth through high school and one for our wedding day. Gardening was another passion of my moms. You could more than likely catch her outside pulling weeds around her several beds of flowers or picking vegetables to share with the neighborhood. Mom loved frogs, our yard was always filled with frog statues and figurines, and there was even a little tiny one that sat on the dashboard of the car. Reading was probably her most enjoyable passion. She loved the Janet Evanovich books, especially the Stephanie Plum serious. I eventually myself got hooked on them thanks to her. I remember mom sitting in the chair all curled up with her blanket, cigarette and coffee laughing until she almost peed her pants. I would give her a funny look and she would read parts of the book to me. If mom wasn't face down in a book or flower pot she had to be sick! My mom didn't like confrontation of any sort. My brothers and I took advantage of this any. All three of us younger siblings pushed her buttons any chance we got. We knew we could get away with more around her than dad. My brothers and I always asked mom first, knowing she would say yes. If we asked dad and he said no. The boys and I went behind dad's back to mom. I have no idea how she managed to keep her cool, which makes her a saint in my book. Let's face it, seven kids in one house six of which were boys, we were assholes. But Tina loved every single minute of it. My mom loved kids period. One of her professions was working in the library in my home town, just shy of ten years I do believe. During the summers mom helped with the summer reading program for all of the kids in our community. She then went on to work in one of the neighboring towns schools as a Para educator to work with kids who had special needs. Those kids meant the world to her. I heard stories about them on a daily basis. Tina was a beautiful woman with very pretty hazel, almost green eyes, very petite and tall, long black, insanely thick, curly hair. Most of the time it was dyed a different color. I remember mom always wearing make-up wherever we went. I used to tease her about it, I would tell her she would put make-up just to take out the garbage... And she would! I always wished I had fingernails as long and pretty as hers; they were always polished and filed perfectly. Mom's appearance was always important as her first real "big girl job" as she called it was as a cosmetologist. I must say people thought my mom was weak and a push over including me, but looking back it was the exact opposite. It takes a very strong person to handle what my mom did, still smile, know when to walk away and keep your mouth shut. I hope to be just like her someday.

Rayleigh and I patiently awaited their arrival; well Rayleigh wasn't so patient, as not many three year olds are. The drive for them was a long one with not much to look at and it was all highway. I lived in the Quad Cities at the time and my parents lived down by Springfield IL. Rayleigh and I set up their beds, made sure we had plenty of clean towels and toiletries. I took my daughter grocery shopping later that morning to stock the apartment with food, munchies and drinks, Damon loves to eat. He can put away some food! Ray had to get all of her new toys and dolls out to show off. I am not sure which one of us was more excited.

I finally got the call from my mom later that afternoon that her and Damon had arrived and needed to be let in. I lived in a locked complex at the time. Rayleigh and I walked down the short flight of stairs to say our hellos and help carry in the luggage. To my surprise we had an extra visitor; my mom brought her Shih-Tzu Rocky. He always was her favorite child. Rayleigh was happier to see him than anyone; they had a special bond since they were born months apart. No one knew Rocky's exact date of birth so we have always told Ray him and her share a birthday. Mom was feeling a little under the weather. Her and my brother almost didn't come for fear of getting Rayleigh and I sick. Since it was my birthday and I had no family close she decided to come anyway.

Mom, Damon and I spent the afternoon catching up on the past month or so. I told mom about a new scrap booking store in town, of course we had to go right that very minute to check it out. Thankfully we did go mom found a lot of military stickers for my Brother Jamie's scrapbook. I guess they are hard to find at the other stores she goes to.

We then decided to head out to dinner at a local Chinese restaurant we referred to as the Die-nasty. It did not have the greatest reputation, but it was good and everyone always ate there any way. We got seated and my mom waited at the table while I got food for myself and Rayleigh. She then went up to the buffet and got her usual salad and frog legs. As soon as mom sat down, she reached across the table and put frog legs into Rayleigh's mouth, before I caught on to what was going on it was too late.

"Was that what I think it was?" I asked.

"Yep!" Mom said with a smile. "They're good Ashley, you should try them."

"Well I guess I have to now that you made my kid eat them!" I was pretty disgusted. I swear it took me ten minutes to get the courage to try them.

"Just try them sis." My mom was laughing at me.

"You know they are pretty good." I said after trying the tiniest bite I could possibly get into my mouth.

"See, I have been telling you for years to just try them. They taste like chicken don't they?"

Oddly enough they did taste like chicken. I had tried something I swore I would never lay a finger on all thanks to my mom, and I actually liked it. You know, mom does know best even though I hate to admit it. We finished up dinner and headed back to my apartment. When we got home my mom did what she does every single year for us kids, bake a cake. Even in my twenties I still got a homemade cake. Mom was a decent cook for the most part but that woman could bake like no body's business! Candies, cakes, cookies, and breads, you name it she made it and it was phenomenal! Every year for Christmas mom would make huge trays of goodies for each of us kids to take to our teacher's. Every one of our teachers had a love hate relationship with mom during this time of the year, but who could blame them? I want to share a recipe of hers with you all so you can enjoy it as much as our family and friends did.

Crisp Peppermint Patties

1 cup of butter flavored shortening

1/2 cup of sugar

1/2 cup of brown sugar

2 eggs

1 pkg of peppermint patties

1 tsp. of vanilla

2 1/2 cups of flour

1 tsp. of baking soda

1/2 tsp. of salt

Cream the shortening, brown sugar and sugar. Beat in eggs, vanilla and melted patties. Then mix in the rest of the dry ingredients. Refrigerate mixture for 30 minutes.

Then drop spoonfuls onto baking sheet and bake at 375 degrees for 8-10 minutes until the tops of cookies start to crack. Recipe makes around 5 dozen.

Later that night mom really started to feel horrible she was coughing, had a high fever, and the aches. She had the flu! Awesome! I went to the store, conveniently it was right across the street and got some thera-flu, tea bags and honey for hot tea and got her tucked into bed. Tina slept well that night considering. The next morning Damon woke up with the same symptoms, even more awesome! I did not get to see them often, so I was pretty upset their time with me was going to be spent with their heads in the trash can or laid up in bed. I spent the day bouncing between mom, Damon and my daughter. I made lots of soup, poured out tons of medicine and tried to keep Rayleigh entertained. I was pretty exhausted and very happy to finally lie down in bed. About 3:00 am that next morning I woke up freezing to death, or so I thought. I sat up in my bed and my whole entire body hurt. I was covered in a sheet, blanket and a comforter I should not have been cold to say the least. I thought to myself, you have got to be kidding me. Off to the bathroom I went to check my temperature and sure enough 103.7, I had the flu! The dreaded flu! I took some Tylenol and crawled back into bed. The next couple days were rough; Rayleigh was the only one who managed to avoid the nasty bug. Damon and I eventually got better, mom did not. I figured she had pneumonia or bronchitis and told her to go see a doctor as soon as they got back home. Mom called me the day after they arrived back home, sure enough it was bronchitis. She was prescribed antibiotics for a few days and told to rest. After about a week or so of her taking the medicine mom was feeling at least somewhat normal again, but I noticed that the cough was still there and pretty rough sounding. I didn't really think too much of it, the antibiotics needed time to work completely and they affect us all differently. Mom finally felt 100 percent, for a day or two anyway and then the cough came back. She called me to tell me she was sick again and would probably be sleeping a lot, not to be worried if there was no answer when I called. I instructed her to call and set up another appointment that maybe the doctor needed to try a different antibiotic, clearly the first one had failed. Mom went back to the doctor. It was the same scenario, went to the doctor, got medicine, felt well after a week or so and the cough came back. At this point I knew something bigger was going on. I called to talk to her a night or two later and she sounded awful, worse than before.

"Mom you need to go back to the doctor, you clearly do not have bronchitis." I was worried.

"There is no point sis, they won't do anything any way."

"Well mom what did your chest x-ray say?" I never heard the results.

"What chest x-ray?" Mom sounded confused.

"Are you kidding me?!" I asked, I was pissed, she was joking right? "You mean to tell me that you have been into the doctor's office twice complaining of chest tightness and a persistent cough and they did not bother to do a chest x-ray?"

"No they didn't, were they supposed to?"

"Well mother you were on antibiotics for bronchitis that obviously did not work not once, but twice. So yes any doctor with half a damn brain would have ordered a chest x-ray." She knew I was furious!

"Calm down Ashley it's okay."

"No! It is not okay. You need to schedule another appointment and demand that they do an x-ray. You are the one paying them NOT the other way around."

Jesus! I am sure that I had steam rolling out of my ears at this point! I am in the medical field by profession; I do not claim to know it all but this is common sense stuff... and a doctor of all people! I called Damon and told him to take her in to the doctor if he had to tie her up and throw her in the trunk of the car. Of course, my mom refused to go. The next day I got a call from her, I could tell she was upset or scared. I was not sure which, but something was wrong.

"Hey momma, what's up?"

"Don't be mad at me sis." She was clearly scared, her voice was shaky.

"What's the matter?" Damn it just tell me!! Of course I didn't say that but I was thinking it.

"Well, the coughing has gotten worse and my left shoulder is starting to hurt pretty badly."

"Okay, well you should have let Damon take you into the doctor."

"That's not all Ashley." She paused. "I am now coughing up blood." Mom sounded like she was going to cry.

"That is it! You're going to the doctor if I have to drive down there and take you myself." By this time I had moved from the Quad Cities to just north of Bloomington. I was only an hour away from her, so she knew I would!

"It's not a big deal sis. I probably just pulled a muscle in my shoulder and broke some blood vessels in my throat from all of the coughing I have been doing." She was trying to wiggle her way out of going to see the doctor and I was not having it.

"Uhm, no Tina it is a big deal! You are not supposed to be coughing up blood. That is not normal. You need to go be seen that way the doctor can make sure nothing major is going on with you." This woman was a pain in my ass sometimes!

"Does dad know about you coughing up blood?" I asked.

"No." Of course dad didn't, if he did mom would have already been sitting in the doctor's office!

I called Damon and told him what was going on and that he needed to take mom in. Under no circumstances was he to take no for an answer and to call me as soon as they were finished. About two hours later I received the call from mom.

"Well I was right, broken blood vessels and a pulled muscle in my shoulder." She didn't sound too sure of the diagnosis.

"Well... What did they do?" Hopefully a chest x-ray I thought to myself.

"More antibiotics and muscles relaxers for my shoulder, the doctor said I still have bronchitis."

BULLSHIT!!!! I did not believe it for one single second!

"Did they rule everything else out which a chest x- Ray?" I have no idea why I even asked, I already knew the answer!

"No x-ray." Mom got silent, probably waiting for me to blow a gasket.

"Are you fucking kidding me mom!?! Did you ask for one?"

"Yes but they said there was no reason for one."

"Oh my god! I'll call you back." I did not even give her the chance to say goodbye or answer back. I just hung up on her to call my dad. I explained to him what mom had told me. Dad said that he would talk to her and try to figure out what to do next. He knew something was not right either.

The next morning on 6-13-12 I woke up to about thirty five missed calls and text messages from my dad and Brother Nathan telling me to call them back as soon as possible. I knew something was wrong so I called my dad back immediately.

"What's going on?" I asked

"Your mom has been admitted to the hospital; the doctors did a CT scan and found a 6-7 centimeter mass on her left lung. The doctors believe it is one of three things, Tuberculosis, Leptospirosis, or..." He paused. "Cancer."

"Wow" I was speechless "What happened? Why did you have to take her back in?"

"She was complaining of pain in her shoulder, was unable to sit still, has barely slept in two days and is still coughing up blood. I told her we go in the easy way or my way." obviously dad was not taking no for an answer.

"Okay where are you guys at? I am going to head that way"

"We are in Taylorville waiting to be transferred to Springfield. The doctor wants her in a negative pressure room just in case it is not cancer and one of the other two."

"Okay, well let me know if you get transferred before I get down there." I am pretty sure I made it down there in record time. I will not come out directly and say I was speeding though.

Just as I was getting into Taylorville dad called me to tell me that they were on their way to Springfield, her room was ready. He told me that they would meet me at a local store there in town. Now I am curious at this point, why would an ambulance pull over in a parking lot to wait for me? Logically with my mom being suspected of having two communicable diseases, I assumed they would transport her by ambulance to keep her from possibly infecting the public. Wrong! They sent mom to Springfield in her own personal vehicle to infect the world. I was not too happy at all, strike one. To top that off we arrive in Springfield at the hospital to let them know that she is here and I notice neither her or my dad have masks on. Strike number two! Dad and I got mom up to her room and then I notice she still had her IV in her arm, uncapped, open to the world! The nurse comes in a few minutes after we arrive with an IV bag in hand.

"What are you doing with that?" I asked. I was extremely nice at this point just caught off guard.

"I am going to hook this up to Tina." The hell she was!!

"No you are not." I said.

"Yes I am. It is just fluids for her she is very dehydrated." The nurse snapped back, Strike Three! Now I am mad!

"No you are not! She has been out in public with that IV port in her arm, uncapped might I add. You will not be hooking anything up to that. You will be taking it out and putting a clean sterile one in."

"I will just clean it off with an alcohol pad and she will be fine." she said as she proceeded to open her alcohol pad.

"If you want to keep your job ma'am, I highly suggest you go out there and get a STERILE one before you hook anything up to my mother's arm, Thank you!" Damn I was irate, who does that?

A few minutes later she returns with the supplies to put a new IV in mom's arm. She was not happy at all but I did not care one single bit. I watched her like a hawk to make sure she was not taking any of her anger out on my mom. I imagined her jabbing mom's arm on purpose just to get back at me.

"Everyone in this room needs to go out into the hallway and get a mask on or they need to leave and wait in the waiting room." The nurse snapped, now that I have pissed her off she is all of the sudden concerned with everyone wearing masks.

"I have been with her all day and not one single person has told me that I need to have a mask on. So why the sudden concern?" My dad snapped back

"She is suspected to have two very contagious diseases and to avoid it being spread everyone needs to be wearing…" Dad cut her off.

'I have been with her in an enclosed room since 3 o'clock this morning. I am pretty sure whatever it is she may have, I am probably infected with it as well. No one was concerned when we were at the other hospital, nor did neither of you care when I had to bring her in my own personal vehicle and risk infecting the public because neither of you offered an ambulance service for her and it was not an issue when she walked the entire length of this hospital without a mask on. But now it's a big issue. This would have been a nice thing to know from the get go."

"I am sorry but we require masks." The nurse walked out of the room.

Now I know we all probably should have had them on, but at this point we had all been around her for an extended period of time, so really what was the point? The logical thing would have been for us to wear masks when we left the room being that we were all exposed and not the other way around. Then again who are we?

Our next run in with super nurse came a few hours later, in Taylorville mom was on 15mg of Morphine and two 5/325 Norcos. Her medicine had been changed to just one Norco and Tina was in a lot of pain but would not tell anyone. The squirming, wiggling and grimacing gave it away pretty quickly. I called the nurse to bring mom some extra pain medicine to help make her more comfortable. I pushed the call light.

"Yes, may I help you?" Ugh it was her!

"My mom is in a lot of pain and I noticed that her pain medicine has been decreased. Can you please get it changed back to the way it was before? It seemed to really work for her."

"I have an order for one or two Norcos I can bring her another one in."

"Thank you that would be great. Mom said to tell you she does not want the Morphine, it makes her to sick. She wants to try just the Norco."

"I will let doctor know and will be in shortly with that second pain pill." The nurse said.

Well that was a lot easier than I had expected it to be. Wrong! Forty five minutes go by. Now I am a patient person especially since I work in the medical field and I am aware of how insane it can be to try to juggle everyone's demands on top of what you are normally supposed to get done. Mom was one of four patients on the floor at the time and there were two nurses. The reason I know this is the nurse was complaining about how bored she was since the floor was so empty that day. There was no reason what so ever for her to have to wait that long. Mom's friend Lorie, who herself is a nurse, showed up not to long after that. I was explaining to her what had been going on in the middle of my explaining she reached over and pushed the button for the call light again. Lorie spoke to the nurse and asked again for pain medicine. Thirty more minutes went by; I was mad and had to go outside to get some air before I exploded into pieces, getting myself kicked out of the hospital. I exited the room and guess who is at the nurse's desk playing a game on her phone? I had to walk away before I jumped over that desk and knocked her out of the chair. I was going to go outside, take a breather and come back up to the desk and politely as possible inform her of what a worthless excuse for a nurse she was. I stood out there ten minutes maybe, as I passed the desk super nurse was gone. Upon entering mom's room I came face to face with the nurse, pill cup in hand, and Lorie smiling from ear to ear. I waited for the nurse to leave.

"Soooo.... What was that all about?" I was sure I already knew the answer.

"I went out to the desk and stood there until she got off of her lazy ass and brought your mother her pain medicine, I had enough!" Lorie said

"That's why I had to leave, I was getting mad. I can understand if they were busy but there is no excuse for this." I said

"I know I went out there and she started to get a little rude with me and I informed her very quickly that I am a nurse and I know how the show is ran and to get your mom her pills."

Thankfully that nurse's shift was over not to long after that. The next few days were nerve racking they took mom in to do a Bronchial Biopsy to test for cancer. The hospital staff had us all wait in an extremely tiny sitting area, my Aunt Missy, dad, Damon and myself were all there along with a few others who stopped by to say hello. We were cramped and thankfully the biopsy went very quickly. I am not sure how much longer I could have sat in there; I was claustrophobic and anxious about mom. After a few hours the doctor came into tell us that mom's biopsy went very well, they were just finishing up and everyone would be able to see her shortly.

My brother Nathan came to see her later that day. He brought her a Chicago Cubs balloon, she hates the cubs. He got the middle finger for that one and probably his ass kicked if mom were able to get up out of bed. It was a good laugh and that is exactly what everyone needed.

Blog entry from Tina June 14th, 2012-

Family and friends, I want to thank you all for the prayers being sent my way. I am very sore and very tired. Not getting much sleep with all the pain that I've been having, as you all know by now, I was admitted to the hospital Wednesday afternoon. I've been having problems with my left shoulder and was told it was a pulled muscle. An x-ray and CT scan was performed and showed a mass in my left lung causing the problem. A bronchoscopy was done and samples of the tissue were taken, we should have an idea in the next few days on what is going on. You don't know how much it has meant to me to hear all of the comments and prayers being said for me and my family. I thank each and every one of you. I am truly blessed to have each and every one of you in my life. God bless you all, Tina and family

June 15th, 2012 a day not a single one of my family members will ever forget. We were all in good spirits until a team of doctors walked into the room. They were straight faced, prepared to deliver bad news. My heart sank I could tell it was not going to be good.

"Well Tina and family we have the Biopsy results back and unfortunately it is not good news." The doctor said.

"Cancer?" Mom asked.

"Yes cancer, you have what is called Adenocarcinoma. It is a very rapid growing, aggressive cancer.

"What can we do?" My dad asked

"We have to wait for them to stage the cancer and we can go from there." the doctor said.

Wow, cancer! You always think that these kinds of things will never happen to you or your family. It did not seem real, they were just kidding right? The whole family was in tears, hugging and asking why? I just stood there, at the moment I felt nothing, numb, as if I were in a bad dream. I finally came to realize what I had just heard; it took all I had to keep from bursting into tears. I knew I had to be strong for my mom. Being in the medical field for almost ten years has made me an emotional robot if you will. We are taught to show no emotion around families. I had a huge inner battle with myself, I wanted to curl up in a ball right there on the hospital floor and cry until I went to sleep, but at the same time I couldn't cry. Not in front of mom. I got on my phone right then and there and did some research on Adenocarcinoma, I had never heard of it before, I assumed since mom was a smoker that is what caused her cancer. Adenocarcinoma is linked to radon exposure and smoking, although it is common in nonsmokers as well. This type of cancer makes up about 40% of lung cancers. From what I saw online her survival rate looked extremely grim.

I left the hospital to go pick up my brother Damon, he was at home and had no idea yet. I was half way to the house when it hit me like a ton of bricks. My mom, my best friend... cancer. Millions of questions ran through my head. Why her? Will she make it? Will she die if so how long does she have? I could not even being to imagine how she must feel. What was going through her head, she must be terrified. How could she not be?

I made it to my parents' house in one piece, still in tears, Damon was upstairs sleeping when I woke him up he looked up at me.

"Mom has cancer doesn't she?" He asked.

"Yes buddy she does." I hated being the one to have to tell him that our mom had cancer.

We both lost it, standing there for what seemed like hours hugging and crying, crying and hugging. Damon and I grabbed a few things from the house for mom and headed back to the hospital. When we arrived the team of doctors was back in mom's room. More bad news? How much worse was this going to get?

"We have staged your cancer Tina; you are at a stage 3. I am so sorry but it is inoperable, it has spread to the lymph nodes surrounding your lung. We can try chemotherapy and radiation but this type of cancer usually does not respond well to it." The doctor said.

"So how long are we talking as far as life expectancy?" My dad asked trying to fight back tears.

"About three months, I am so sorry Tina. If you have any questions or there is anything at all we can do for you please let us know." The doctors left the room.

That's it? We only have three months left with her? Why? She took the news very well. Better than anyone else took it; she was the one telling all of us not to cry. Mom was going to beat this, her determination was unreal. Tina sat there in the bed head held high. You would never have known she was just told you only have three months left to live. I was so proud of her and the outlook she had. I did not expect a bright future for her at all. I made a call to the Red Cross to get my brother Jamie home as soon as possible. He was serving in Afghanistan at the time. The doctors and nurse we had that night did an amazing job working with the military to get Jamie back here to be with mom. We only expected him to get a furlough. The military allowed him to come home for good and be released of his orders overseas. We were going to have to wait a few weeks to see Jamie though; he had a reintegration period he had to go through once back in America.

Mom came home that next day, still with a great outlook on her tragic news. Tina did not let this keep her from doing what she loved, the scrap booking and gardening continued as they always had.

Blog entry from Tina June 17th, 2012-

Thank you everyone for the prayers and kind words. I am home from the hospital and getting settled in for the ride of my life. We should find out more tomorrow as I have my first appointment with the oncologists. I also want to thank my bestie for just being you and for the bath and body works assortment. They will come in handy in the near future, Jamie M. for the YUMMY roast, my friend Carla for the beautiful roses, my sister Chris and 3 beautiful nieces for the beautiful flower arrangement. To our kids for everything you have done to make coming home easier for me. I love you all very much and am so very blessed to have each of you in my life.

A few days passed, Tina went to her first oncology appointment at the cancer treatment center. A game plan for treatment was discussed, with operating being out of the question the doctor was going to have to try to attack this with chemotherapy and radiation only, in hopes that alone could do the trick. The day after the first appointment with the oncologists mom received a phone call that made us all jump for joy, there was a light at the end of the tunnel! Her cancer was not a stage 3 it was a stage 2 and contained to the lung. The cancer was not in the lymph nodes as they doctors had originally thought. They were going to be able to operate! Thank you Jesus! Thank you! Thank you! Thank you! She had a fighting chance. The doctors set her up with aggressive chemotherapy and radiation treatments for 5-7 weeks. Radiation was Monday through Friday and chemotherapy on Thursdays; surgery to remove the tumor was to follow at a later date.

Blog entry from Tina June 19th, 2012-

Now that Jamie is in the loop I can and will share with everyone. First appointment with oncology went well. PET scan showed a few more spots of cancer cells that appeared to be on the outside of the left lung, which is why I was staged at a level 3 cancer. We were explained in detail what the plan of attack of treatment would be, WELL FORGET WHAT I JUST TYPED, YEAH!!!! Shortly after returning home, phone rings and it is my oncologists. He and the cancer surgeons, YES I said cancer surgeons, consulted over the test results. The new spots that were detected are on the inside of the left lung, which means the cancer is contained to the left lung, which in turn puts me at a stage 2 cancer. I was crying and couldn't even tell Bryon. All I could do was pass the phone to him and tell him it was the doctor. Thank you all for the prayers and PLEASE keep them coming. God is hearing our prayers. My family and I have a long hard road ahead of us. I'm strong, stubborn, and ready to fight.

I recall mom spending the day on the phone with family and friends cheering, laughing and crying. She had been kicked harder than she had ever been kicked before; this news was just what she needed to help push her to fight even harder. Later that night there was a knock on the door. There stood a young man who our family had known since the day he was born. He himself had battled cancer, not once but twice. Around the age of three he was diagnosed with leukemia. I can remember going to a few appointments with Alex and how heartbroken I felt seeing not only him, but all of those babies fighting for their lives with so much life left to live. Watching all of those kids hooked up to machines, tubes and receiving chemo, or ladybugs as Alex called it, just makes you want to trade places with each and every one of them. He beat his cancer only to be diagnosed again. This young man fought again and beat it twice! Truly an inspiring human he is!

Blog entry from Tina June 19th, 2012-

Tonight I received a very special gift. A young man that I have known since the day he was born has battled cancer twice in the 13 years he has been on this earth. He brought over and put on me his prayer arrow that he wore during his last round of chemo. He said it helped and he now wanted me to have it. Talk about tears rolling. I love you very much Alex.

This young man was secretly my mom's inspiration. He has been through more than any young child should ever have to endure in their life. That day meant so much more than words can describe to my mom. That prayer arrow proudly hung around her neck every single minute of every single day.

The following week seemed to drag for everyone. We anxiously awaited Jamie's arrival home. It had been months since any of us had seen him. The occasional phone call or video chat was the only communication we had with him. Seeing his face was long overdue!

Blog entry from Tina June 24th, 2012-

HE IS HOME..... Thank you JESUS!!!!!!!!!!!!!!!!!

Jamie being home was more than exciting, for mom it was bittersweet. Ninety five percent of her days were spent worrying about him. I remember her pacing back a forth, not even realizing she was doing it. If mom had not heard from him in a few days she was ready to call the Red Cross, the president of the United States and any other person who she could get a hold of to make sure he was okay. My mom and dad threw a small get together in their back yard to celebrate Jamie's return from overseas. If I had to pick who drank the most amount of alcohol out of everyone, I am not sure if I would be able to do so. That night was quite entertaining to say the least.

Mom's next appointment came and went. The doctors scheduled her for surgery to have the port for chemotherapy put in and the first chemo treatment was immediately after.

Blog entry from Tina July 18th, 2012-

OK family and friends. Need prayers for tomorrow. I have to be at the hospital early for the placement of my port. Once out of recovery from the surgery I go straight to my first chemo treatment. Bryon, the kids and I all want to thank all of you for the support that you all give us on a daily basis. You have all made this battle so much easier than it ever could have been. Your daily meals, phone calls, text messages, cards, and house visits mean the world to us. We will never be able to repay you all. God bless all of you! Bryon, Tina and Family.

If there is one good thing about living in a small community of 900 people, it would have to be the massive amount of support and help you receive, whether you want it or not. Everyone lines up to bring over meals, food cards, gas cards for appointments, anything and everything you could possible think of or need. In some sense it was the community battling the cancer right alongside mom.

The first few days of mom's chemotherapy and radiation went very well. Everyone commented on how good she looked for being on chemo. Right around the forty eight hour mark is when it hit mom and it hit her hard, the vomiting and nausea wiped her out. I took as much time as my job would allow so I could be there to help her. I arrived to the house one day, mom was hugging the toilet and greener than I have ever seen anyone before.

"Hi." She muttered

"Well hello there beautiful, how are we doing?" I asked

"How does it look like I am doing?" Mom said as she flipped me off, at least she still had some spunk in her.

"You look like hell, I still love you though. How has your pain been?"

"Not too bad, I thought I was going to be okay with this chemo. It hit me all of the sudden this morning and all I have been doing since is vomiting. I guess forty eight is the magic number."

"Have you been able to eat anything at all?" I asked.

"Not since last night, the thought of food today is making me sick."

I helped mom back to the recliner and got a bucket to cut down on the trips to the bathroom since she was so exhausted. I hated watching her vomit over and over, knowing there was absolutely nothing in this world that I could do to stop it. A pat on the back and saying it's okay mom just did not feel like enough. I can't recall a time in my life where I felt so helpless and useless. How can I go to work each and every day, knowing I help other people get well and go home but I can't make this any better? I even went as far as questioning my ability to be a nursing assistant. I broke down and told mom how I felt.

"You know mom, the hardest part about all of this for me is going to work and being able to teach my residents how to function again at home and watching them leave, but I can't do anything to help you."

"You are good at what you do sis. I am proud of you for what you have done. You can't win them all honey. I used to laugh at you because you brought every stray animal home with in a five mile radius and tried to save them. I always knew you would do something that involved caring for people or animals and I really am proud." Damn she was right, again, as always. This was different she was the person who gave me life. Cancer really does suck.

All of mom's time was consumed with appointments. Every single day of the week, except for the weekends she had to be at the hospital for chemotherapy, radiation, doctor's appointment or random combination of the three. It started to take its toll on her and fast. Within the first week mom had lost four pounds from vomiting and lack of appetite. The doctor decided to add another nausea medication to the list in hopes it would stop some of the vomiting. Over the next week Tina's appetite slowly increased, trips to the bathroom were fewer and fewer. The medicine was doing its job.

Blog entry from Tina July 26th, 2012-

Day 2 of trying to eat myself to death! LOL I love when meds actually do what they are supposed to do. 2nd round of chemo went well.

Weighed in and I have gained back 3 of the 4 pounds I lost. I fixed a mini picnic to take with me, and slept for about an hour of the treatment. Tomorrow is my last radiation for the week. Pray and keep your fingers crossed that I stay nausea and vomiting free so we can head to Harvard this weekend for Bonnie and Clyde's (AKA Lucy and Dylan's) birthday party. Again thanks to all of you for the thoughts, prayers, tests, phone calls, meals on wheels and everything else. I am truly blessed to have each and every one of you in my life. God has been good to me by bringing you here. Take care and HUGE ((((HUGS))))!

Mom's weight slowly started to rise as each day went on. It was nice to see her want to eat a meal, enjoy it and keep it down. Her energy levels rose as well, vomiting takes a lot of you. Even through all of the sickness there was still a smile on her face, it was a forced smile I am sure, but there was one there. Everyone noticed a change in her just over the few days she was on the new medication, it was apparent the nausea medication was a total success. This medication could not have been introduced to mom at a better time, just a few days afterwards on August 4th 2012, the villages of Buffalo and Mechanicsburg, where my dad was employed as a police officer put on a benefit for my mom in the park in Mechanicsburg. The weather could not have been more perfect. The sun was shining with not a cloud in the sky, not to hot, not to cold, around 80 degrees or so. The benefit was set off early that morning with a poker run, they even brought the parade of people right in front of my parents' house, honking and screaming to show mom the support she had. Her eyes teared up; she was truly grateful what was being done for her. When it was time to leave for the benefit we had a convoy of several cars all sporting our new Tina's Troops window stickers to escort mom. Nathan took his semi that was proudly decorated with flags, cancer ribbons and a huge flag that said Tina's Troops that all of the grandkids painted for her. Tina's Troops was a slogan our community quickly adopted to show mom their support, t-shirts were made by my dad's friend Scott for everyone to purchase and wear at the benefit. The shirts were all grey, they had a black silhouette of a dove flying through a white cancer ribbon and "Tina's Troops" written in big letters across the back of the shirt, the design was awesome. When we all arrived to the park there were already more people there than we had imagined. People came from all over to help support my parents. Tons of activities were set up for every one of all ages, the biggest hit being the smoke house for the young children. Mom got a huge laugh watching them dive and roll from the windows. The face painting booth was a close second; puppies, lions and butterflies roamed the park. Right after a barbeque lunch of hotdogs and hamburgers the fire departments set up a mock car accident. Almost everyone there gathered around to watch the men and women use to Jaws of Life to extract dummies from the beat up car. I personally am a trauma junkie so this by far was my favorite part of the benefit. Immediately after the accident was a truck and car show. Several muscle cars, motorcycles, trucks and semis entered. My brother Nathan entered his semi into the show and won the title of "Best Truck". I am not sure who was more proud, him or mom. I think he carried the trophy around with him the entire benefit. Over all the silent auction was the biggest deal. Several places donated some really neat stuff and everybody wanted them. We had roughly ten to twelve tables full of photo sessions, massages, toys, gift baskets of lotions and candy, gift cards, gas cards, Major league baseball tickets and the most popular item being the hood of I believe it was Dale Earnhardt Jr.'s race car. Over $6,000 was raised for mom just from the silent auction, which did not include other donations made. Tina was beyond shocked and felt truly blessed so many people cared about her enough to give their own hard earned money to help her out with medical expenses.

Blog entry from Tina August 6th, 2012-

I have no idea where to start, but here it goes! I knew I was blessed but I guess I never knew how much until this past weekend. I want to start by saying thank you to three very special people, Sam for having the idea and taking it to Mary Lou and Jodi, who hit the ground running with it. You are truly angels here on earth. My benefit was a success. I enjoyed visiting with each and every one of you that were there. If you weren't able to make it believe me I could feel your presences there with me, giving me strength. I hope everyone had a wonderful time visiting, eating and catching up with some friends of years passed. I want to thank Scott for making the t-shirts. We still have orders coming in. To the rest of the Mechanicsburg fire, EMS and police departments, THANK YOU THANK YOU THANK YOU!!!!!!! This would have never happened without all of you. Last but not least my friends and family. To my hubby, you have been here by my side through this whole rollercoaster ride, and at times it has been just that. I love you more than life itself. To my children and babies, you are my world. Always have been always will be. You are my heart! To my BFF, you are the best. 48 years of friendship WOW! I love you Belle! To everyone else, I thank you, Please keep the prayers coming they are still needed, God bless you all! Tina

Mom was overjoyed from the amount of support from the benefit. Things for her seemed to really be looking up, until she noticed that her hair starting falling out. She called me one night in tears.

"It's falling out sis." Mom said.

"Is it bad?"

"Not yet but I washed my hair tonight and I noticed that the bathtub started to hold water, I took my foot and rubbed it across the drain and there was a huge clump of hair down there."

"Are you going to shave it off like you said you were?" I asked.

"No it isn't bad enough, but when I brushed it a lot more came out in the brush, I just sat on the toilet and cried."

I felt so bad for mom; luckily she had enough hair for six people so it was not noticeable at all. The next week on August 18th mom, dad, Jamie, Damon and Jamie's girlfriend Nikki all came over to celebrate Rayleigh's 4th birthday. Ray was on cloud nine that her mawmaw and pawpaw were there and had brought her a brand new Barbie bicycle. Mom and I baked a cake and let her decorate it herself. It was quite the masterpiece and had enough icing on it for several cakes. Tina enjoyed watching her open all of her presents from everyone and Rayleigh said it was her best birthday ever! She got tons of new dolls, adorable clothes, a giant horse and doll to match, way too much candy and money. Her favorite present by far were her two new rabbits, actually seven new rabbits. One of the rabbits happened to be pregnant when I bought it; we walked out in to the garage to find five little rat looking animals all over the floor. It was not until I saw rabbit fur all over the place that I realized what they were. Unfortunately none of them lived, the mom abandoned them all. Later on the evening we lite a fire and had some drinks outside. Before mom went to bed she yelled for me to come into the bathroom.

"Ash can you come help me for a minute?"

"Yea, what do you need?" I asked.

"I need you to help me put some cream on my burn." She said.

I walked into the bathroom and mom was standing there in front of the mirror with one arm out of her shirt. I could see the radiation burns on her shoulder blade and collar bone. I cringed just looking at it. I have never seen a burn that bad before in person; her skin looked fake and was raised about a half of an inch. The blisters were extremely large and starting to bust open, the area around the wound was very red and warm to the touch. The whole entire wound was a little larger than a soft ball. Her shirt was covered in dry, flakey skin chunks. Too my surprise it did not hurt her as much as I thought it did. I rubbed some silvadene cream on the burns for her.

"Does it hurt?' I asked.

"Yea a little but not as much as you would think, my clothes are what bother me the most, especially bras, the straps sit right across the burns."

"I would be peeing my pants, it looks awful. Did the docs say if it would scar or not?"

"There is a possibility that it will, I don't care either way. It is in a spot that no one is going to see it." Mom said. She always thought positive.

The next morning maw maw and paw paw went back home so mom could rest before her next set of treatments. Tina was joyful her treatments were nearly over. I could tell she was beyond ready to be done with the daily trips into town. Mom felt like the chemotherapy and radiation were consuming her life, and they were. Everything had to be planned around her treatments. I know Tina felt like this was a burden on everyone, time and time we told her it was not. I am sure I would have felt the same exact way if I were in her shoes. It had to be done and none of us minded switching things around to help make life easier for her. This particular week was joyous week for mom it was her last radiation treatment.

Blog entry from Tina August 23rd, 2012-

Well I am done with radiation WOOHOO!!!! That is until surgery. Two more large doses of chemo before surgery also, they are possibly looking at mid-November for surgery. Thanks for all the prayers and please keep them coming. I've only covered 1/3 of my journey. I am truly blessed to have each and every one of you in my life. Don't know how I could have made it without all of you, God bless each of you! Tina

Once Tina finished her radiation the doctors decided to do two larger doses of chemotherapy before her next pet scan. After the first dose she really started to lose her hair. It was extremely noticeable when she had her hair up in a ponytail. Mom had to wear her hair down in order to cover the larger bald spots right above her ears. I know how self-conscious she was about the hair loss. Especially the week of her second treatment, she went into visit all of her kiddos from school. This was the first time mom had been in there to see everyone since the diagnosis. It worried her what the kids would think seeing her like this but thankfully it went very well.

Blog entry from Tina September 12th, 2012-

It was wonderful going into work on Monday and seeing all of my co-workers and the kiddos. I miss you terribly and can't wait till I can return to work. Thanks again to all of you for the cards, prayers, money and best wishes for my recovery, I'm very proud to say I work with the most awesome group of people! RES rocks!!!

Tina's treatments were coming to an end, she did okay with them for the most part, considering. The two big doses are the ones that hit her the hardest. It was getting harder for mom to do the things she once loved as weakness was setting in pretty hard by this point, I can remember her teaching my two best friends and I how to do gymnastics in the front yard. She was not able to do these things anymore and would miss out on doing them with all of the grandkids. Although a lot of joy came from watching them all play, it was not the same and she missed out on so much. I wish I could have taken it all away from her! Mom really started to lose her hair, this time it was extremely noticeable. It was falling out in huge chunks and mom was devastated, before it was easy to cover up. She finally gathered the courage to let Jamie shave her head bald. I recall her calling me in tears, extremely upset, but there was a sense of pride in her voice. Mom was going to wear that bald with pride and did just that.

"It is gone sis, I did it." Mom said

"You will have to send me a pic, I want to see. I will shave my head with you if you want me to." I was curious how she looked.

"No you will not and I will kick your ass if you do. Your hair is so long and you have been growing it out forever now and I don't want you to cut it." Said Tina

"You're worth it mom and it will grow back, I think we should all shave our heads with you. It shows that we support you."

"You can support me without buzzing your head Ashley."

There were several agencies who gave mom wigs to wear; one of them in particular looked just like her natural hair, as if she had never lost it all. Although she did not wear the wigs ever, mom hated them actually. They made her head feel disgusting. I know it must be hard for a woman to lose all of their hair, especially hers it was so long and beautiful. Tina finally adopted the motto bald is beautiful, it was a look that she pulled off well. I again offered to shave my head with her and played with the idea if just doing it anyway but she really would have kicked my ass! My mom was one of the few people I was scared of so I listened to her.

Blog entry from Jamie October 2nd, 2012-

Just buzzed moms head... She cried most of the time.... She looks good bald thought! Love you momma!

Once mom's hair was all gone we sat down as a family and explained to Nathan's four kids and my daughter Rayleigh that grandma was not just sick as we had been telling them, that she had cancer. Nathan's older two knew exactly what was going on and they understood what cancer was. The younger three we had to explain to them in detail what it was and what happens. This was by far the hardest part so far. How do you explain to young children what cancer is and make them understand? How do you find the words to tell them that grandma may pass away? There is no easy way to do so. The kids were hysterical as you would expect them to be. As hard as it was there was a sense of relief for me, I had stressed since the day I found out mom had cancer. How was I going to tell my child? I was very happy to have everyone there with me to help. We explained to the kids that they were going to have to be more careful with grandma and keep their toys picked up since mom was becoming more unsteady. We did not want her to trip and fall over them. In hopes to lighten the mood a bit mom promised the kids the next time they came down for a visit she would have finger-paints on hand and each one of them would get a turn painting her bald head. Their tears suddenly turned into giggles and frowns turned to smiles. Mom defiantly had a way with kids. Each one of us children had to step up and help as much as possible when we were at the house. I am sure I speak for everyone when I say how incredibly proud of all of the grandkids I am. They all helped mom get the things she needed, such as food or water. They all did and amazing job playing quietly when mom needed to rest. We truly have amazing children.

Blog entry from Tina October 3rd, 2012-

Family and friends tomorrow is my last chemo treatment WOOHOO!!!! No more poison for a while. Thanks for all the prayers and PLEASE keep them coming. I still have a long road to recovery.

After several weeks of chemotherapy and radiation mom was done! It is mind boggling what five to seven weeks on a medication can do to a person. The day of her last treatment the doctors set up and appointment for the 10th of October to do another CT scan to see if the tumor had shrank any. I don't think that any of us were very optimistic as her initial prognosis was not very promising. It felt like all we had received was bad news. To everyone's surprise the treatment had worked, and better than we imagined! It was dead and half the size from when she started treatment. All of us jumped for joy. This was a true miracle; mom had gone against all odds and beat this! A total dream come true. The doctor and surgeon decided to push forward with surgery to remove the mass. We could not have been happier, how mom must have felt. The next few weeks were celebrated with phone calls to family and friends. She had beaten this monster. Her faith, drive, ambition and tons of support pulled her through.

Blog entry from Tina October 10th, 2012-

Praise God from whom all blessings flow!! Just back from the doctor, the tumor is has shrank to half the size it was and is dead!!!!! Just waiting to hear the date for surgery to get the damn thing out of my body. Thank you all for the thoughts and prayers. God is AWESOME!!!! Please keep them coming as I am on the last leg of this journey. I don't know what Bryon, the kids and I would have done without all of you. Bless you all, Tina

The surgery was scheduled for a month later on November 13th, 2012. Joy and feelings of sorrow were mixed between the family. We knew mom had beaten the cancer but she was not out of the woods yet. The toughest part was still to come. I knew she was weak from the chemotherapy and radiation, my concern was her being strong enough to go through surgery. Tina's spirits were higher now than I had seen them in a very long time. Through the treatment, even though she kept her faith there was a sense of fear she tried to hide. That was now gone, my mom was back to herself.

Mom and dad came up for the weekend, right before mom had her surgery. Rayleigh for some reason was scared of mom's bald head. It was not grandma is what she kept telling us. After several failed attempts to get Ray to touch or kiss mom's head we finally had success.

"Monkey you know what I heard?" Mom said

"What?" Ray asked bright eyed

"Well, the doctors told me that if I want my hair to grow back I have to have a little girl kiss the top of my head." Mom looked over at me and smiled

"No way, not me!" Said Rayleigh shaking her head.

"How will my hair grown back then if you won't kiss my head?" Mom pretended to cry.

"Okay grandma, don't cry. I will kiss your head for you." Ray reached up with her little hands, brought mom's head down and kissed the top of her head. I had just enough time to snap the cutest picture I have ever taken in my life.

"Thank you Monkey." Said mom with tears in her eyes.

"Why isn't it growing back yet? It didn't work!" Rayleigh asked very disappointed

Giggling mom said "It worked honey. Hair grows really slow so you will not be able to tell for a while."

For weeks upon end Rayleigh told everyone she saw that her kiss would make grandma's hair grow back. We even started a trend around town. My parent's neighbor Patty was diagnosed with ovarian cancer shortly after mom was. She went through chemotherapy as well and when Patty lost all of her hair, she did the same thing with her granddaughter. I was deeply saddened that someone else so close to our family was going through the same mom was. In some sense I was relieved mom had someone she could talk to who understood what she was going through and dealing with since none of our family had ever endured the pain she was experiencing.

October 20th 2012 was a day mom had a very hard time with. My brother Dan got married and she was unable to attend because her immune system was too weak and physically mom was unable to travel. I know it broke her heart that she had to miss it while all of us kids were there. It was a beautiful Catholic wedding. I had never been to a Catholic wedding the ceremony was very long, which I was not used to. I can honestly say I have never been so moved at a wedding, the music and the church were absolutely breath taking. My sister-in-law Megan was stunning. The flower girls had the most adorable skirts made out of tool and they wore leotards underneath. I made sure to take tons of pictures to show mom. Dan's and Megan's reception was held at a country club tucked off in the woods in Wisconsin. The happy couple had an open bar for the first two hours of the reception; needless to say everyone was drunk within those two hours! Other than one mishap I had a great time, it was nice to be able to see and spend time with all of my brothers. I think the hardest part for mom was that this was the first time in thirteen years that all seven of us kids had been together in one place. We fulfilled mom's one request and took a picture with all of us at the reception, one goofy and one serious. They both turned out great. Mom received a copy of it from Nathan and hung it on the wall right by her chair so she could look at her children anytime she wanted to.

The day mom had the upper lobe of her left lung removed was frightening but bittersweet all in the same sense. It was an early morning for us all, especially mom and dad. They had to be there to register mom and fill out the mounds of paperwork you have to sign beforehand. Shortly after the staff took Tina up to be prepared for surgery and all of the family went into a large waiting room just outside of where mom would be. I was happy to see the reclining chairs because mom's surgery was expected to take several hours. My dad, Jamie, Damon, Aunt Tammy, mom's cousin, her husband and Lorie were all there to support her. All of us were in a great mood, this was a great day! Tina was having the cancer removed from her body for good. Everyone laughed and joked while we anxiously awaited her return. My brothers even played jokes on my aunt. The best one by far was when Jamie kept putting a subscription for AARP into my aunt's purse. I don't know how many times she threatened to beat his ass. I think my aunt Tammy may have a secret fear of aging! None the less it was hilarious. Everyone shared stories of mom, the main one being her complete lack of a sense of humor, which tended to be the topic of conversation a lot in our family. No one knows how she missed out on the funny gene. We are loud mouthed smartasses to the fullest. Tina was the black sheep and missed the crazy train by a long shot. I can remember times growing up when dad would mess with people, whether it be at the store or a restaurant and everyone would get a huge kick out of it expect for Tina. She always scolded us for being inappropriate or rude, no one cared she was mad because it was always so funny.

A few hours passed and the receptionists in the waiting room called our family to let us know that the doctors were coming to speak with us. Everyone was panicking, it was way too soon. Something must have had to have gone wrong; there was no way they were done already. Those ten minutes it took for the surgeon and doctor to walk down from surgery felt like years. Fortunately they delivered great news, mom made it through surgery like a champion. Tears of joy filled our eyes, the surgeon was able to remove all of the cancer and the radiologists placed radiation beads in her chest wall to kill off any cells they may have missed. The doctor did deliver some not so pleasant news; there was a very likely chance that this cancer would return. Just when we thought that this was all over, we got kicked in the face. The battle for mom may not be over. Everyone just had to be strong and hopeful that it did not show its ugly face again. The doctors said mom was in the process of being moved to a recovery room and we would all be able to see her soon. Dad and I went down there first. I must say she looked great for just having one of her organs removed.

"Hi momma how are you feeling?" I asked. She lifted her right hand and wiggled her fingers, which meant. I am feeling with my fingers. This is something my grandfather always used to say.

"Smartass" I laughed "You're still high aren't you?"

"Very much so." Mom said with a little smirk

Blog Entry from Ashley November 13th, 2012-

Mom is out of surgery!!!!! She did well; we are just waiting for her to wake up. Tumor was attached to her aorta and radioactive seeds are in to kill any leftover cells.

I left and went back to get Jamie and Damon so they could all go see her. Everyone made their rounds into the recovery room. After a few hours the staff took mom into her room on the pulmonary unit. The boys dad and I all went and had lunch while she got settled in. We came back up and there were tubes, wires and monitors all over Tina's body. The worst one of them all being a chest tube to drain the fluid off of her lung and chest cavity. The surgeon had to go in through mom's left side; her ribs had to be separated so the lung could be reached. Thankfully the nurses were amazing and kept on top of her pain medication so she could relax a little bit.

Blog entry from Tina November 13th, 2012-

Day 13.....Today I am thankful that we KICKED CANCER'S ASS!!!!!!

Everyone took turns staying the night with mom at the hospital so she didn't have to be there alone. The next few days were a repeat of the day before, nurses came in to check and drain her tubing and catheter, check her vital signs and deliver pain medication. Respiratory therapists worked with mom to build up strength in her lungs and gave nebulizer treatments. Surprisingly mom's lung function and oxygen levels were amazing and right where they should be.

Blog entry from Tina November 15th, 2012-

WOOHOO!!!!! Chest tube is out!!!!

On the fifth day post-op mom got to come home. A lot of changes had to be made, everyone had to step up and do their part to make sure the house ran smoothly. Tina was unable to do any lifting at all; although she wanted to I am sure. I helped mom with her baths, I had to help her undress, get in and out of the shower and wash the right side of her body because she was not to use the left side at all.

Blog entry from Tina November 20th, 2012-

I know I haven't been keeping up with my thankfulness list, but just had to write today. Day 20.... Today I am thankful that I had lather when I shampooed my hair tonight. Yes I said hair! It is finally starting to grow back. It is very fine, but by golly it is there. I am also thankful for my daughter running the homestead while I am down. Belle I am thankful for you always being there when I need you. Thanks for staying with me my first night in the hospital. I don't think that either one of us slept with all of the snoring going one LOL. To my cousin, you have been a God sent for me. God bless you my cuz and I know he will. Most of all today I am thankful for every one of you that throughout this journey has brought in a dinner, donated to my benefit, came sat with me, called to check in on me, or just sat in your house thinking of me but couldn't bring yourself over cause it made you cry to think of me LOL. You know who you are and I love ya, ya redhead!!!! I am thankful I am getting a bit stronger every day. Still hard to breath at times and I have shortness of breath a lot, but I am alive and able to enjoy thanksgiving with my family and friends. God bless us all and NEVER pass a chance to tell your loved ones that you love them. Tomorrow isn't promised. I love you all and God bless. Tina

I know that this made mom feel helpless, things she once did for herself were ripped out of her hands. Independence was always mom's strong suit, do it herself rather than ask others for help. She wasn't even able to use the bathroom on her own.

Not long after the surgery was Thanksgiving. Mom and dad came up for a few days. I attempted to cook my very first Thanksgiving dinner. I made turkey, green bean casserole, corn, mashed potatoes, sweet potatoes, cranberry relish, cranberry sauce and no Thanksgiving dinner is complete without pumpkin pie. Dinner was surprisingly a success, I did not burn the kitchen down, the food was good and no one died. I was so proud of myself. Mom even told me how proud of me she was, which put a huge smile on my face. Following dinner was our traditional food coma nap, which I am positive every American partakes in. The rest of the night was filled with movies beer and even a small bonfire. It was the perfect night to sit outside around a warm fire and roast marshmallows. I could have sat out there forever, that moment it felt like nothing was wrong in the world. Everyone was happy and talking about old times, not a mention of mom's cancer. My parents left the next afternoon after lunch. Rayleigh and I were sad to see them go; I was more at peace with them leaving because mom seemed to be getting around a lot better than she was.

A few days after my parents returned home mom had scheduled an appointment with her doctor because she has having a lot of pain and tingling in her left side, especially her foot and hand. I remember the phone call very clearly mom seemed upset she had another new medicine.

"Hi momma what are you doing?" I asked

"Oh, I just got back from the doctor, I am pooped." She sounded very tired.

"How did that go?" I asked

"I have another new medicine, the doctor said the cause of all of my numbness is neuropathy, I have to take Gabapentin now."

"Hopefully that helps; I know it was causing you a lot of pain. You have to be careful with it though it can make you dizzy."

A diagnosis of neuropathy was given. He said it was in fact from the surgery, and it may never completely go away. The doctor prescribed Gabapentin, which is an analgesic and has shown a decent success rate in treating neuropathic pain due to cancer. Tina was not too thrilled to add yet another medication to colossal list she already had. Mom would always joke that she was a walking pharmacy. This diagnosis qualified mom for disability which was a huge help since her and dad did not have health insurance. Mom filled out all of the paperwork and sent it in. After a few weeks she received a letter saying her disability was denied. My parents were not happy about this at all being that mom met all of the qualifications for this service. They got in contact with an attorney to see what steps needed to be taken. Most of the time people get denied on their first attempt, so mom filled out the paperwork for an appeal, which she won. Her disability had been approved. So many doors were opened with this approval, so we thought. Mom and dad were under the assumption that mom's medication would be partially covered since she now had insurance. In order for the medication to be covered they had to pay a certain amount out of pocket first. The amount required out of pocket was more than their monthly income. To me this made absolutely no sense. How do you expect someone to pay more out of pocket than what they bring in? The excuse given was that my dad has a good job. There is some truth to this but regardless of the fact that he has a good job, they were required to pay more than he makes. My parents were stressed enough as it was, just when they thought there was some hope they got shot down. My major problem with this entire issue is my parents have both worked their entire lives and paid their dues as far as taxes go and never used any sort of help from any agencies. Now that they are in dire need of it mom gets turned down. Is that not what it is there for? People who need it? I was beyond furious, as I see this happen with my job all too often and personally it makes me sick to my stomach. Families are stressed enough due to the fact that our economy is crumbling at our feet; let's just throw more sand in their eyes! After this whole ordeal I noticed that mom's prescriptions, especially the pain medicine, had more pills in the bottle than what should be in there. She had been taking half doses or simply skipping them all together. Her thoughts were if she could make a months supply last two months it would be less of a financial stress on her and dad. This is one of the few times I recollect hearing my parents fight, my dad was not happy that she was sitting there in pain. He stressed to her not to worry about the money and to take her pills like the doctor had prescribed.

The month of December seemed to fly by everyone seemed to cherish this Christmas more than before. We had mom with us and she was supposed to be gone by now. I don't think I have ever felt more joy during a holiday. It was a very small get together with the family; the only things that were missing were all of mom's goodies she used to bake in years passed. Mom was doing much better but still wore out and tired easily from the surgery.

New Year's rolled around and Rayleigh went to her dad's house in Iowa to celebrate Christmas with them. I got to spend a little extra time on the phone with mom. She was very cheerful and excited to see a new year, although mom did not make it until midnight. That was not like her but what she had just been put through in the past seven months I cannot say that I blame her for crashing early.

Blog entry from Tina January 30th, 2013-

OK it is official..... CONGRATS to my hubby on his promotion to Police chief of Buffalo/Mechanicsburg police department. I love you honey. Congrats to Sam also for making sergeant!

This promotion could not have come at a better time; dad received a decent raise as well, helping relieve some of the financial stress from the medication and doctor bills. Things were finally starting to look up for my parents and our whole family at that. Mom was doing much better, her hair was growing back in curlier than before, dad got a promotion, and life was good.

A week or so before my mom had her three month checkup Damon and I went together and got tattoos in moms honor. We both got cancer ribbons that said "For my hero" underneath. There was a slight variation between the two, the left side of my ribbon was cascading hearts that got bigger the further down they went and in the middle of the very bottom heart mine said "mom". Dear lord was mom pissed when she found out!

"Why in the hell would you put that junk on your body? I just don't understand it." She screamed when I told her.

"Just wait until you see it before you get your panties in a bunch, they are really pretty."

"I doubt it!" she said

I will never forget the look on her face when she saw them. Tears immediately rolled down her cheeks.

"I love it, I hate tattoos and I love it." Mom said

"I told you that you would like it." I said smiling. I did not expect her to cry.

"This means a lot to me that you two did this for me."

A month or two prior my Aunt Tammy went and got the same tattoo except hers was colored in purple and said "sister". We tried to talk Jamie into going with Damon and myself but I think he was too much of a chicken to go.

In February mom went into the doctor for her three month post-op checkup. A PET scan was performed and we were delivered with wonderful news. Tina was three months in remission, she was still cancer free! Things were looking better than ever, everyone was ecstatic. The fact that mom really may have defied all odds and truly beat the unbeatable made everything seem perfect.

Blog post from Tina February 21st, 2013-

Good report at the doctor today. CT scan is showing two areas that are scar tissue. Doctor feels that this and the neuropathy are the reason for all the pain I am still having. He also gave me the ok for Bryon and I to head out west this summer to see my sis! WOOHOO!!! Thanks for all the prayers. I will see the oncologists on March 4th. Let's pray for a great report from her also.

Tina's Sister Chris lived in Utah and invited my parents out there for a few weeks in the summer to visit. All we heard about was how mom could not wait to get out there to visit. I don't believe they had anything set in stone at this point; details were to be worked out at a later date. Mom was doing well; things were finally getting back to normal for her. Sundays were filled with races on T.V. Rayleigh learned to tie her shoes on her own, using the bunny ears trick mom taught her. There seemed to be not a care from anyone. All of our routines went back to normal, work, school, daycare and family time were what they had been before mom got sick. I felt relieved I did not have to worry about mom and how she was doing. Each day she got stronger and was able to do more and more on her own. Even with the neuropathy Tina seemed to push through and do whatever she had to do to build up her strength.

May 5th Mom's dad Merle had his 75th birthday party and fish fry in Salisbury. He had the same party every year in the same place; this would be the last year he did it. The turnout was pretty decent although I did not know a lot of the people there. My Aunt Missy brought her baby Olivea who was the life of the party. Everyone wanted to hold her because she was so stinking cute. Lunch was very good. Mom had me try a piece of what I thought was fish.

"Here sis try this fish, it is better than the other. I am going to have to ask dad what kind it is." Clearly I have not learned my lesson with the years of frog leg torture.

"That is really good; find out what it is please. I would make this at home." I said

Mom burst into laughter. "I know exactly what it is Ashley."

"What in the hell did you just feed me!?" I could not spit it out because I had already swallowed it.

"You don't want to know." She said in tears

"Yes, yes I do want to know!"

"Testicles, you just ate pig testicles."

"You bitch! I really don't like you right now and I will never trust you when it comes to food again." I wanted to gag, that is disgusting!

Mom was proud of herself she had tricked me and I fell for it again. She made her rounds to all of the family laughing telling them what she had just done to me. Of course every one of those sickos agreed with mom that they are good. I have to admit they did taste good but that was not the point, I just couldn't get over the fact that they were part of an animal's reproductive system, just plain disgusting!

Memorial Day weekend came around it was a gorgeous day outside, perfect weather for a cookout. Usually it rains so we were all happy to have such great weather. Mom, dad, Rayleigh and I went to Jamie's girlfriend's grandmother's house for a cook, and out. We all had lots of laughs because Jamie had a hard time figuring out the grill. His manhood was questioned quite a few times during the grilling process. We even discovered Grandma Judy's yard was full of poison oak, thankfully no one caught it. After a few hours of being there my cell phone alerted me that Sangamon County, the county mom and dad live in, was under a tornado warning.

"Hey dad did your phone get any weather alerts?" I asked

"No why?"

"Well mine just popped up and it said Sangamon is under a tornado warning."

"No I got nothing it is probably just a glitch in the system." Dad did not seemed concerned; he is usually on top of the weather so I did not worry about it. About twenty minutes later Jamie came outside.

"Uh dad you guys may either want to head home now and fast or shack up here for a while, we are about to go for a ride. The radar is nasty and there are tornado warnings all over the place.' Jamie said.

Dad reached into his pocket and grabbed his phone. He played with it for a few moments and looked up.

"Tina we need to head for home. It is getting pretty nasty." Dad said

"Why don't we just stay here until it has passed over?" Mom asked

"We have time to get home if we leave now, but we need to go."

All four of us loaded up into the car and headed back to mom and dads. The drive all through Decatur was clearly and sunny, not a cloud in sight, which was eerily odd since the storm was supposed to be fairly close. Dad drove other ten miles or so and noticed the clouds rolling in. We were about a half of a mile from home when it hit like a ton of bricks. My father is not scared to drive in storms; he reached over and turned the radio off so I knew it was bad. Rayleigh was in the back seat talking ninety miles a minute as she normally does. I asked her to be quiet but she continued to talk. Just before I could yell at her dad chimed in.

"Enough Rayleigh!!" He screamed at her, she knew he meant business

"I am sorry." She said as she started to cry.

"I am sorry Rayleigh this storm is bad and I need to concentrate so I don't wreck I need you to be quiet." Dad's voice was shaking, I really knew now it was not good.

I could feel the car pulling in different directions as the wind and rain slammed against the side. I thought for sure that the car was going to flip. The rain was not coming straight down it was swirling in circles around the car. You could not see the lines on the road in front of the car it was raining so hard. I was worried about debris hitting the car because we would not have been able to see it until it came shattering through the window.

"Are we caught in a freaking tornado dad?" I asked, more like yelled it was so loud.

"I am not sure, but I think we might be." He said, He was struggling to keep the car on the road, or what he thought was the road.

I have never been caught outside in a tornado before, nor do I care to ever be again.

"Oh my god!!" mom screamed as we pulled up to the house.

"What?" Dad asked

"It is gone, the fucking tree is gone!"

"Holy shit it is!" Dad said.

My parents had a sixty to seventy foot fern tree in their back yard and the storm had cut it completely in half.

"Alright everyone when you get out of the car run like hell to the house." Dad said

I got Rayleigh out of her car seat and wrapped her head up in my arms and took off out of the car. The wind was knocking my feet out from underneath of me. I had one hell of a time trying to get to the door. Once I got into the house I put Rayleigh in the bathtub with a pillow and blanket from mom and dad's bed and went back outside to help dad get mom into the house. She was struggling more than I was. Dad and I both grabbed an arm and practically carried her into the house. The power had been knocked out so dad walked to the back door to check the power lines and the back yard looked like a war zone. The fern tree had fallen onto the other larger tree my parents had in their yard and knocking part of it over. The bottom part of the fern tree was resting on moms swing. There were power lines, branches and debris scattered all over the block.

Dad had a family friend of ours, Jimmy, come over to help trim up all of the branches so the power company could get the lines back up. Jimmy barely got a start on the trimming when he fell off of the ladder and broke his ankle. Dad called the paramedics and he was loaded up into the ambulance and sent to the hospital. The day after Jimmy fell off of the ladder mom and I kept smelling something burning, neither one of us could figure out where it was coming from. We both tore the house apart trying to find the source. Rayleigh came running into the living room about an hour later screaming that something was on fire. I jumped up and she took me right to the phone jack. It had shorted out and was now on fire, thankfully it was a small fire and Rayleigh caught it. Lord knows what would have happened if she was not in the kitchen when she was. I am sure we all had enough action that week to last us a life time.

Mom went in for her six month post op checkup and CT scan in June, waiting for the results was nerve racking, she had made it this far in the clear.

Blog entry from Tina June 11th, 2013-

"I am asking for prayers once again family and friends. Well my 6th month checkup was not a good one. The CT scan they took last week is showing several spots in the outer most layer of what is left of my left lung. I am scheduled for a full body PET scan on the 17th and then a biopsy on the 25th. Then back to the oncologists on July 2nd for the results. The doctor said she did not want to guess what was going on, she wants to know for sure. She mentioned the cancer being back as a possibility and if so it is at stage 4 which there is no cure. But it can be controlled with more chemo. She mentioned modules and scar tissue. We all did this once before and I know we all can do it again. Prayer is powerful, and our God is AWESOME!!!!!!!"

The whole family waited patiently for mom to have the PET scan and biopsy done. I am sure the ones of us who never prayed before were surely praying now that it was just scar tissue.

Three days before mom went in for the biopsy I moved back home to my parents' house to give dad an extra set of hands since she was having trouble with her neuropathy. The move was an absolute disaster right from the get go. The rental truck I rented was double booked, I had virtually nothing packed, my apartment almost caught on fire, I was not sure if we were going to make it to the storage unit in time to unload everything before they closed. Thankfully I had tons of people volunteer to help me and the day worked out pretty well in the end. I was glad it was over and happy to be close to mom since she needed someone there. Maw maw was very thrilled to have Rayleigh there all the time. With Rayleigh and I living so far away for all of these years mom did not get to see her but a few times a year, being at the house with grandma and grandpa made Rayleigh feel very important. She got to be grandma's helper, her biggest job being dog duty. Ray had to feed, water and walk Rocky every day. Don't you dare do it for her either, that was her job and she was proud to be helping. Mom referred to Rayleigh as her monkey because when Ray was a baby she used to make a face that made her look like a monkey. Ray had a few other things around the house that she got to do, getting water for mom, helping grandma with her slippers and from time to time she even got to paint moms toenails, I started a full time job in a nursing home about 30 miles away working first shift. I had to leave for work by five in the morning so this meant that Ray got to spend the day with grandma. I loved getting pictures from mom of the two of them playing outside or walking to the library. I'll never forget the day I came home from work to a huge surprise according to Rayleigh anyway.

"Mommy, guess what!?" Ray screamed as I walked up to the house.

"What!?" I yelled back to her.

"Look what grandma got me." She said as she pulled a little blue card from behind her back.

"Oh my! What is that?" I already knew mom had called me and told me.

"It is my very own library card. I can get books all by myself now." Rayleigh was beyond excited.

The PET scan results came back and there for sure were three spots roughly the size of pencil erasers in the membrane around the void where her lung once was. The oncologists decided to go forward with the biopsy. Dad took mom in and the procedure went smoothly and fairly quick. When the results came back everyone was devastated. Tina's cancer was back which automatically staged it at a 4. There was nothing they could do this time as far a treatment; they could only try to contain it.

Blog entry from Tina July 2nd 2013-

"Well as most of you know by now my test results came back positive for cancer, NASTY BASTARD as Paula puts it. This means it is at a stage 4. I will start chemo again within the next 7 to 10 days. I will have to do this once every three weeks with a CT scan to follow the 3rd treatment. I am a fighter and plan on giving this monster a run for its money. Please keep the prayers coming they can only help!"

The doctors set mom up with the first chemotherapy appointment; Tina was nervous but determined as always to fight. Nathan's kids came down to stay a few days before mom started her first treatment. It is never a dull moment when all of the kids are together. They say and do the craziest things! We are on our toes non-stop. Thankfully mom felt well enough at this point to get outside and play with them a little bit. Something she had not been able to do for quite a while.

Blog entry from Tina July 8th, 2013-

"Had a productive day today, played with the grandbabies here at home and at the school park. Came home to find a knot and bruise on Destiny's forehead. She hit the stairs while playing hide and seek with Dylan. Then we get home and Dylan sticks a tiny toy up his nose and can't get it out. Paw paw to the rescue! Love these babies of mine!!!!! Very blessed they are mine!!!!"

This was an interesting day that is for certain. Destiny came running into the living room screaming.

"Grandma! Dylan's nose is bleeding."

"Why is his nose bleeding?" Mom asked while leaping out of her chair.

"I don't know." Destiny said.

"Tell him to come down here so we can take a look at it." Said mom.

Dylan came to mom and sure enough his nose was bleeding. Dad took out his flash light and looked up his nose.

"You have something shoved up there you ding dong." Dad said

"I know." Giggled Dylan.

"Why would you stick something up your nose? Don't put stuff up there buddy you can hurt your big brain." Laughed dad.

Dylan thought it was funny. Paw paw pulled out a very large bead. How Dylan managed to shove that thing up there is beyond me. Having most of the grandkids around seemed to help take mom's mind off of having to go through chemo again. No matter how hard life was for her the grandkids always made her smile and forget about reality, even if only for a short time.

Our family received a great surprise on July 26th, 2013 our old neighbors from down the street came to visit. We had not seen each other in nearly fifteen years, since they moved to Florida. I used to baby sit Pam and Greg's kids, they were all grown up and had kids of their own. Christy brought her boyfriend Jordan and their little girl Sophia, who is an absolute doll. Unfortunately Ryan did not get to come; he had since moved to another state and was busy with his family and work. They stayed most of the day at our house. It was an unusually cold and rainy day for July. The temperature was in the 50's, which was cold to them; they all like to froze to death. We all teased them about being so used to the Florida weather that they had become soft. I then got ganged up on for the time I was babysitting and burnt popcorn so bad Pam could not get the smell out of her house for weeks. I will never forget that, nor do I think any of them will either! The rain finally got to be way to much we had to move inside. The visit with them lifted mom's spirits, it really was nice to chat and visit with people we had once been so close to.

Mom started chemotherapy shortly after all of the company went back home. The nausea and vomiting were a lot worse than the last round. Her doses were much larger than the first set of treatments. This had its good and bad points; good being that mom had more time between treatments to recover and was not sick the whole entire time. The bad however, was bad, right from the get go she was violently ill. Tina's hair fell out again, a lot faster than before. The second time around with the hair loss was not as difficult on her as the first. Mom just took it for what it was. Before each round of chemotherapy mom had to have lab work done to make sure her blood count was stable enough for the treatments.

Blog entry from Tina July 30th, 2013-

"Back from oncologists. Good report today. Blood counts are good so I am in the clear for more chemo next Thursday. Let's just hope I don't have the nausea again I had with the first treatments. On another note, I need suggestions for some high calorie foods that DON'T include dairy. I lost seven pounds, Dr. wants me to fatten up."

Over the next few weeks mom finished up her first round of chemotherapy, the nausea was awful, her weight and appetite really started to drop. Unlike before this time around her weight loss was noticeable. A CT scan was scheduled to check whether the spots had shrunk.

Blog entry from Tina September 16th, 2013-

"Had CT scan this morning to see what the chemo is doing to the tumor. Please pray it is shrinking it and containing it. God is good and his will be done."

My Aunt Tammy came over to visit with mom after her appointment and brought some med pass shakes they give to residents in nursing homes who do not eat, to help with mom's weight loss. Tina was not fond of them at all; she said "They taste like shit." Mom fought through the taste and actually drank them. I have no idea how; the smell alone was enough to make me want to gag. It was a nice visit for mom; she did not get to see my aunt that often due to her crazy work schedule. Of course my aunt gave mom a lecture about not eating and that she needed to keep up her strength into order to continue the chemotherapy treatments.

Blog entry from Tina September 19th, 2013-

"Well as most of you know by now, the cancer didn't shrink, but grew a slim bit. It could have been worse. Got to have that positive outlook! They have taken me off chemo by port and are trying Tarceva which is a chemo pill I will take once a day. They are telling me the side effects from this are less than the chemo I have been taking. Which is less nausea and means I should be able to eat and less weight loss. I should not lose my hair, and hopefully not so tired. I still need prayers as my family and I continue to fight the battle and bump in the road that god has given us. I thank him every day for the blessings I have and most importantly the 2 new little blessings we have coming very soon, Rylan and Jaycee. Thank you for all of the thoughts and prayers to this point, but please keep them coming. They mean a lot and I love seeing all of your uplifting comments. God bless all of you, and I feel very much loved and fortunate to have each of you in my extended family! Tina and family"

The chemotherapy was not affective at all this time. The doctor wanted to take mom off of the chemo by port and switch to a new inhibiter pill called Tarceva. This pill was not actually chemotherapy, it is used to slow the cancer cells only, not kill them. The doctor put in the order for the medication. It would be sent to mom by mail in roughly a week or so, she was to take it once a day. We then discovered this medication was around $6,700.00 per month and the only way insurance would cover it is if my parents had met their total out of pocket expenses for the month, as I said before was more than their monthly income. How on earth do these people expect anyone to pay for something that is almost $7,000.00 a month? Dad was enraged as to be expected, it was ridiculous. My parents were already paying for all of mom's medication out of pocket as it was. I picked up a few for them here and there, the cost of her normal day to day medication was outrageous enough let alone this. Tina got in touch with a counselor at the cancer center and explained to her the situation and asked what could be done. There were several options but none of them looked to promising. The counselor called the pharmaceutical company that made this drug and asked if they offered assistance. They did but only once the out of pocket cost for the month had been met, they then would cover a portion of the cost. This defeated the whole purpose; if the out of pocket cost had been met then the drug would be fully covered. She called several different agencies for mom trying to find a solution with no luck. This meant mom had to go without any treatment until something could be worked out. Mom was devastated and dad was furious. I know they both felt as if there was no hope.

Blog entry from Amanda September 27th, 2013-

"I can't begin to express how much I love children and sometimes little school papers I get at home makes me love them even more! Destiny came home with a paper she had to write explaining what she would do if she had $100.00 to spend. This was her answer. ""I wodu giv my mune to my grama tat haz cansr."" I cried. She is such a kind heart, loving little girl!"

I remember how proud and touched everyone was by this. Kids really are the kindest souls around. We as adults do not give them the credit that they deserve. I know I automatically assume they have no understanding of what is going on. In reality it is the total opposite, they understand a lot more than what we are aware of. Destiny knew that mom was sick; she knew that financially mom and dad were struggling and she understood that they needed the money more than she did. Many children that age would have went on a crazed shopping spree at a toy store. Destiny offered it to her grandparents. Such a smart, kind child she is.

Blog entry from Ashley October 28th, 2013-

"Happy birthday Jaycee!!!! She's perfect!!!!"

Such a joyous day, my Brother Damon's little girl Jaycee was born and precious as ever. She looked just like Rayleigh when Rayleigh was born, it was very eerie the resemblance they had. Mom was beyond excited, her and dad went to the hospital and spent a big part of the afternoon there. Mom raved about how cute and tiny she was. I was jealous I had to work and was unable to go up there until the following afternoon. Once I did make it up there I stole her away from her mom and held her the entire time I was at the hospital. I defiantly developed a case of baby fever, my baby was all grown up and seeing those big fat cheeks made me miss all of the things about a baby, well except the diapers. Becca and Jaycee were only in the hospital for a few days and they got to come home. Of course all of the attention was now focused around the new baby and Rayleigh did not like it. She adored her new baby cousin but hated the attention she was receiving.

Bryon's work puts on an annual Halloween party for the village every year at the police department. It has become quite the little party. As always it was extremely cold outside and the wind was terrible. Thankfully the guys got hay bales to put around a huge bonfire for everyone to warm up around. There are hotdogs to roast and s'mores for later on in the night. EMTs usually judge a costume contest for the kids and then one for the adults, I love seeing all of the little ones in their costumes. The biggest deal of all is the haunted house the guys put on. They spend at least a week setting up for it. Thousands of dollars have been spent over the years on props and dad has received tons of donations as well. We usually have around ten people or so who help out in the haunted house. This particular year my boyfriend Lee and I decided that we were going to go all out. Lee spent a couple of hours online researching zombie makeup ideas, he found tons of really neat ideas that use simple house hold items and food. The morning of the haunted house we both spent four hours doing our makeup. I used oatmeal and liquid latex to make my face look as if I had some kind of gross skin condition. Toilet paper and liquid latex were used on my chin and forehead to give me an aged look. I mixed plain gelatin and liquid foundation and applied it while it was warm and sticky to my arms and neck to look like something had taken huge bites out of me. I think between Lee and I we used about three vials of fake blood, one large tray of cream makeup and two tubes of grey-green cream makeup. I was a zombie nurse and very happy with how well it turned out. My boyfriend's costume was disgusting. He used the gelatin mix, shaved half of his head, and smeared the gelatin all over the shaved spot, his ear and down his neck. It almost looked as if his brains exploded. He used toilet paper and liquid latex to build up a thick layer on his nose and then peeled it backwards towards his eyes to make his nose look like the skin had been peeled away. On the left arm the gelatin was used again from his shoulder to his hand, he made it look as if his entire arm had been badly burned. I have to say this was the most fun I had ever had at Halloween. Lee and I stopped to grab food before heading to the party and about gave the girl at the window a heart attack, she screamed and threw the stuff she had in her hands and ran away from the window. I think every single person at the party complimented our costumes and dad asked us to do the makeup for everyone the following year. The highlight of the night was when the lady in charge of the costume contest came up to us and said that no one had entered for the adult group and handed us over $100.00 worth of gift cards. Everyone who put the party together decided that since Lee and I worked so hard on our costumes that we deserved all of the prizes from every category of the contest. It was a great night for me but I looked over and saw mom sitting around the fire by herself, she looked sad. She was usually a huge part of the haunted house and I know that it killed her to not be able to do it this year. This is something that my family had been doing since I was in junior high school, so over fifteen years. Now she was no longer able to handle it. I know mom was wondering if she would even be around to see next years party. Deep down I felt horrible, this was not like my mom to be so down in the dumps. I hated that she was not able to get up and do the things that she once loved doing, even all of the adorable kids in their costumes did not seem to make her happy either.

Thanksgiving came; everyone in the family did their own thing. Looking back I wish we had spent it together, with mom. Mom and dad went to my grandma's house and celebrated with his brothers and sister. Jamie went to his girlfriend's parents' house to celebrate. I ended up going to Lee's parent's house with him. I got to meet a lot of his family members from Montana. Even though we were not all together everyone had a great time at their different dinners, a big piece of me regrets not going to my grandma's with my parents.

The day after Thanksgiving mom has always put up the Christmas tree. Lee, Rayleigh, mom and myself all spent the day putting up and decorating the tree. I despise that thing! It has to be one of the biggest, fullest, prickliest trees I have ever come across in my life. Each branch goes on individually. Putting that tree up is literally an all-day project but we got it up.

A few weeks before Christmas mom took a trip up to Nathan and Amanda's house to spend a week with the kids. After a day or two there dad gets a call from Nathan, he thinks that something is wrong with mom. He told dad that he posted a picture of her online to go take a look at it. Dad brings the picture into me.

"Look at this!" dad said as he flipped his phone around.

"Holy shit did she have a stroke?" I said. Mom's face was drooped on the left side. Her smile was very crooked.

"That is exactly what I thought, Nathan just called me and told me to look at the picture, He said that she is not acting any differently just that her face is drooping."

"Well it looks to me like she had a stroke." I said. Mom did not feel any differently than she did before, or so she said. I was concerned because I had heard this type of cancer can cause strokes towards the final stages.

I went with mom to her next appointment and talked to her doctor about putting her on Aspirin just in case. The doctor did not believe she had suffered from a stroke and felt that there was no reason for her to be on Aspirin. I questioned her as to why she felt there was no need and explained more thoroughly what had happened with mom. I never did get an answer from her, but who I am anyway? I did not agree with her decision at all, what is it going to hurt at this point anyway, as much as I hated to think that way there was some truth to it. She has been without any treatment for almost a month, in my opinion they did not seem to concerned with her wellbeing anyway or the doctors would not have let her go without treatment for as long as they did.

Finally after over a month with no treatment mom's Tarceva, by the grace of God was covered. We heard a knock on the door; it was the delivery guy dropping off mom's medicine.

"Grandma who was that?" Ray asked

"It was the guy bringing my medicine." Said mom

"Bringing your medicine for what?" Asked Rayleigh

"For my cancer honey."

"Oh, well we should just cancel your cancer." Ray said

"I wish it were that simple sweetie." Said mom with tears in her eyes.

I wish it was that simple to. It is moments like that, when your children say the sweetest possible things ever. It really shows you just how innocent and kind hearted kids really are. Tina took her first dose as soon as it arrived. The rest of that day went very well; the next morning was another story.

"I don't feel right sis." Mom said

"What is that matter?" I asked

"I don't know what is wrong, my heart feels like it is racing. I have never felt this way before and it is scaring the hell out of me. The only way I can describe it is that something is inside of my chest vibrating"

"Do you need to go to the hospital? I can call dad." I asked.

"Yes please call him this is really scaring me."

I called dad at work and he immediately came home and rushed mom into the hospital. Mom had mentioned earlier in the day she was supposed to take the medicine twice daily. I was looking at the bottle and noticed it was prescribed for once daily not twice. I instantly called my dad in a panic.

"Dad I think I know what it wrong with mom, she told me the medicine was supposed to be taken twice a day and it is only once daily. I think she may have over dosed herself on it." I said

"Get the bottle and count the pills, there should only be two missing if she took it once a day."

"There are twenty eight left. Thank god! I saw the label, freaked out and called you."

"Well thankfully she did not take to many. I think we need to take over her medicine from here on out." He said

"You know she will have no part of that what so ever dad."

"I know but we need to try."

Somehow people caught word of it fast and my phone went crazy with text messages and calls wondering what was going on and how mom was doing. Tina was released a few hours later; the doctor thought that is was a reaction to the Tarceva and immediately stopped it. We were back to square one, mom was without treatment again.

Blog entry from Ashley December 23rd, 2013-

"Sorry to anyone that I did not answer earlier. My phone was flooded with calls and messages and I had to answer family first. Mom is okay and home. She had what the doctor's think was a reaction to her new medicine. But she is fine and doing okay! Thank you all for you concern!"

Christmas came the following day for us, I had to work Christmas morning so Santa Clause paid and early visit to Rayleigh so that we could all watch her open her presents together. Ray is such a spoiled little girl. Mom enjoyed watching her face light up as she opened everything that she had asked for. Santa is the best!

A week or so later mom went to stay with her cousin for a few days, this was the start of a new Tina that none of us expected to see. Mom came back from her cousin's house and left straight for my aunt's house for a week. This went on for over a month. At one point she had not been home in almost five weeks. Tina got really distant from all of us. She would barely answer our phone calls or text messages. None of us could figure out what we had done wrong. She was dying and these were the last moments that we would have with her and mom did not want to spend them with us. The final straw for me was when I walked in on Rayleigh crying.

"What is wrong honey?" I asked as I knelt down next to her.

"I don't want to talk about it." Her infamous saying every time she cries.

"Why are you crying? Talk to me."

"I don't know why grandma hates me."

"Raybug, grandma does not hate you."

"Yes she does, she left and never came back, she is mad at me because I don't listen."

I called mom right away, I was not nice to her. I regret this now but at the time I did not.

"What is going on with you?"

"What do you mean sis?"

"Don't sis me mom, what did we all do to piss you off? You are dying and you want nothing to do with any of us. I switched my whole schedule around and left a shift of co-workers I love so that I could be home with you and you have not been home since. Now your granddaughter is sitting on the couch crying because she thinks that you hate her. So what is going on? What did we do?"

"Nothing let me talk to Rayleigh."

I handed the phone to Rayleigh and what mom said to her next pissed me off even more than what I was before. Who was this woman?

"Now why on earth you would think that I hate you?" Mom was not talking to her she was screaming at her. Rayleigh started to cry again.

"I don't know because I don't listen." Ray said

"I don't hate you at all now stop thinking like that." Mom was still screaming.

I have never hung up on mother until that moment. I was so frustrated and furious with her. I called my dad and told him what she said. We both agreed that something was going on with her and assumed the cancer had moved to the brain or that mom was having strokes that we were not aware of; regardless of what it was something had changed in her. Her voice was different; she did not care about anything at all. Mom was very unsteady on her feet and was forgetful. I called my Aunt Jenny to talk to her about how I was feeling, we had a big disagreement. We both took what the other said out of context, ending in a huge screaming match. Thankfully we said our peace and apologized fairly quickly. We defiantly did not need that on top of what was already going on.

In the beginning of February my Aunt Jenny called my dad to tell him that she had spoken with this cousin that my mom had been staying with. This cousin was bad mouthing my mom and told my aunt that she thought my mom was making all of her symptoms up for attention. That mom liked everyone waiting on her hand and foot because she was lazy. Boy, did this start a war. Jamie and I both sent this cousin nice long messages about what a bitch and horrible person she was, we both thanked her for taking my mom away from her family in her last days to only turn around and crush my mom's feelings. This cousin of hers did a lot for our family in the beginning and was someone that my mother became very close to and loved dearly. For this person to say such things about mom absolutely crushed her, mom cried for days she was beyond hurt.

I know people have their ups and downs but my mother was nowhere near lazy and hated the fact she was unable to do a lot of things for herself. We did not hear from this person again after Jamie and I sent messages.

Blog entry from Bryon February 7th, 2014-

"Tina does not get on here very much due to her illness; we received bad news we were dreading to hear today. Her time left is short. She has fought through this, to try to beat it. She has kept her faith which is more than I can say. She is blessed with tons of people who have helped her keep strong. She is the love of my life."

Mom had a doctor's appointment on February 7th 2014 and did not receive good news at all. The doctors were done, there was nothing else that they could do to help mom. They were going to put her on hospice. This would not have been so hard on mom had the doctor not have told her "Well it has been nice knowing you." After this day my mother lost all of her will to live, and who can blame her. What else is left to fight for when the doctors tell you that there is nothing else that they can do. Mom had still been having a lot of problems with her heart. When we received her last PET scan results back we found out why. The Tarceva was not what was causing her A-fib, the cancer had taken over mom's entire body. There was a very large tumor that was pressing against her heart cause her heart to spasm. The cancer had taken over mom's lungs, liver, kidneys; her entire chest wall was full. There was another tumor that had wrapped itself around her spinal cord and made its way up into her brain. At this point the doctor was thinking mom only had a few weeks left with us.

Blog entry from Ashley march 22nd, 2014-

"I have tried to be strong through all of this, keep my composure and emotions to myself. Be tough for my mom. Driving home from work this morning it was all I could think about and I just lost it. Being in the medical field you learn to keep your emotions in check but it is so much different when it is your mom. It is so hard to look at her because the person I see is not my mom. She does not look, talk, sound or act like the same person, almost a stranger. I feel helpless because my job is to help people. I help rehab and send home dozens of people a week and I cannot do anything to make this better or make it go away. I am finding it hard to be strong. Watching my mom suffer is the hardest thing I have ever had to do. She is truly my hero, taking on 4 kids, my brothers and treating them as her own. Being the rock that kept us all together when we should be falling apart. When I needed her at 3 am because Rayleigh was sick, she was there. She has always been the better person in any situation. People say bad things about her and she still smiles in their face and talks to them like they are her best friend, which I know I could never do! I wish I could take this all away!! I love you mom!!"

Tina really started to go downhill; it was getting hard for her to even walk. A few times mom fell, unhurt thank God. One day I walked into find her climbing over the coffee table, because her leg rest was in the way.

"What in the hell are you doing mom?" I scared her to death.

"I have to go to the bathroom."

"Okay, but that doesn't explain why you are half on the coffee table."

"Well sis I can't rely on you guys for everything. I have to do these things for myself."

"Mom, when in the hell have you ever climbed over the coffee table? Do you want to break your neck? Because that is where you are heading!"

"I guess you are right." She said as she climbed down.

"Walk around Tina Jesus!"

I got the middle finger, but only because mom knew I was right!

Blog entry from Nathan March 23rd, 2014-

"Ok friends, I normally don't put too much stuff about what is going on, on here. But this is the best way to get everyone's attention at once. My mother Tina as some of you may know was diagnosed with lung cancer and is going to be starting home hospice soon. She is at my house now visiting with her grandbabies. Nothing could keep her from seeing her grandchildren. She had a doctor's appointment Friday and was told that her battle with this monster of a disease is nearing the end. It is very painful and heart breaking to watch someone that is very near and dear to your heart to go through something like this and you can't do anything about it. She is by far one of the strongest women I have ever known. Still looking out for others and making sure they are doing okay. We are going to be having a get together on Sunday the 30th at the mini mall on 5th street in Illiopolis for whoever wants to stop by and see Tina. It would be great for her to see everyone. She is doing well while she is here for the week visiting the babies. She is watching the race right now. But please if you get a chance on Sunday even if it is only for a minute or two it would mean a lot. Thank you all for your support and prayers. I love you Tina, you have meant more to me than I could ever put into words, and you are my angel!"

After talking with mom, she decided that she did not want a whole bunch of company at the house, she just wanted to rest. We decided to hold what we thought would be a small get together for her at the min mall on the other side of the block from their house so that everyone could come and see her at once. The get together exploded with people. We were shoulder to shoulder in there. We had people come that we did not know to show mom their support, tons of friends, family and a lot of mom's former classmates came to see her. There were a lot of tears and hugs from everyone; it was hard to see such a strong woman so frail and weak. Our friends Bill, Deloris, and Nancy set up and donated everything for the party. My brother Danny even drove down to see mom which was a nice surprise we did not think that he was going to make it since his schedule is always so crazy. Everyone took tons of pictures with mom and brought her gifts and cards with money. This was beyond what any of us ever imagined it to be. Mom said that sometimes she felt alone in this journey, this showed her that she was far from that. After about two and half hours mom was done, she was wore out, sore and tired. There were still people coming by to see her but she just could not keep her eyes open anymore. The few people that did stop by after mom left were close friends of the family and were able to come by the house to see her. I know that mom said she did not want the company but you could tell just by the look on her face that she enjoyed it.

The next day mom started hospice, the nurse came out and assessed her. Surprisingly her vital signs were still perfect, although mom sounded terrible. Her lungs were starting to fill up and you could hear her wheezing all of the time. We talked mom into getting a hospital bed and oxygen just in case she needed them. The delivery guy came a few days later and set them up for her. Mom took a great liking to the new bed; she had not slept in a bed since her lung was removed.

Mom had a very nice surprise shortly after starting hospice, our family friends from Oklahoma came down for a short visit. My mom was thrilled to see Carla but so tired she did not get to spend much time with her. I know it was hard for Carla to see mom like this but she felt she had to make one more trip to see mom. She and mom were very close friends and she did not think she could ever forgive herself had she not come. Mom really tried to fight through the sleep; she was not very successful at it. Carla told mom not to worry about it and to just rest. Right before they left Carla and I had a long talk about the past, how we wished this had never happened to her. We both knew the battle was over, stood out on the porch hugging and just cried. I know she did not want to leave, if it were possible for her to stay with mom until she passed that is right where she would have been.

The next visit with the nurse was a pain. She went through all of moms medications with me and told me that I would be taking them over. I was fine with this because mom had not been taking them like she was supposed to be. She now was taking way more than what she was prescribed or just plain forgetting to take them. I was unaware of how much she was actually on since mom had been doing them herself up until this point. Mom was on Tylenol #3, Norco, and Ibuprofen for pain. Ativan and Zofran for nausea, Trazadone, Melatonin and Ambien to help her sleep, Gabapentin for neuropathy, Dilitazem for her A-fib, a laxative and stool softener. I have no idea how she kept them all straight, which was scary.

The following week when the nurse came I expressed to her my concern about mom's pain and all of the pain medication that she was taking. I found pills that mom had hidden from me and was taking on top of what I was giving her. I told the nurse that what mom was taking was not strong enough and that we needed to figure out something else to give her. The nurse discontinued the Tylenol #3, Norco and Ibuprofen and switched to 5 milligram of liquid morphine and a 25 milligram extended release morphine pill. Mom had been complaining the Trazadone was not helping her sleep, it was only making her feel anxious, so the nurse told mom to stop taking that as well. I spent the night cleaning out all of mom's old pills and putting in the new ones. After the first week mom was on hospice I was beat. Rayleigh was still in school, I was still working full time third shift hours and mom required a lot more care. I started sleeping on the couch next to her in case she needed something I was right there. I know that mom was afraid to be alone so she did not let me sleep much at all. It felt like she always needed something, little things and it was starting to wear on me. I loved my mom to death but let's face it she was driving me insane! I would fill up her cup with lemonade for her, start to doze off and she would wake me up for more. She was chugging it so I didn't fall asleep on her. The bathroom breaks of course became more frequent. I could not keep up with her.

Nathan and Amanda came down to visit for a few days, Amanda was a God sent taking most of the load off of my shoulders so that I could actually go into the other room and rest. I have no clue what I would have done if they had not come to visit. Dad was working during the day which left me with mom and while I was at work during the night time hours he was there alone with her. Neither one of us were getting much sleep at all so it was nice to get a full night of sleep. Amanda actually got mom to eat something while she was down, which is something mom had not done in a few days. The day Nate and Amanda left the nurse came back to see mom, her vital signs were still great but mom had lost a significant amount of weight and was becoming more restless, especially at night. The nurse decided to up mom's dose of liquid morphine to 10 milligrams, double her Ambien to 10mg and wanted me to start giving the Ativan twice a day now instead of once daily. Nathan and Amanda went back home, dad and I jumped right back into taking care of mom around the clock. The medicine change seemed to help but only for a few days. I had to take time off of work to be there with mom. It was getting to be too much stress on me and dad was not able to take off of work since mom's bills were racking up. The first few days of being off of work were nice, I did not feel as stressed, but that quickly changed. Mom had a very apparent stroke one night that took out her whole left side; she had no use of it at all. We were now doing everything for mom because she was so weak to begin with and now losing use of one whole side of her body made it impossible for her to do anything on her own. Dad called Nathan to tell him what was going on and he and Amanda came back down for a few days to see her, we did not expect her to make it through the weekend. Mom's breathing slowed tremendously she became somewhat unresponsive. I decided to tell Rayleigh that grandma was going to pass away soon, she lost it.

"Come here for a minute Raybug I want to talk to you." I said.

"What mommy?"

"Well sweetie you know that grandma is very sick right?"

"Yes, she has cancer."

"Yes she does. Do you know what it means when someone passes away and goes to heaven?" I was not sure how to do this. I've never explained death to a child before.

"Yes it means that they will go live in the sky with God, my daddy told me that."

"That is right honey. Here very soon grandma will be going up to the sky to live with Jesus." She started bawling. "It is okay bug; grandma will always be with you in your heart."

"I don't want her to be in my heart, I want her to be on the couch where she always sits." This made me cry.

"I know baby me to. I wanted you to know that way if one morning you wake up and grandma isn't here you will know why okay."

Thankfully Uncle Nate and Paw paw took over from here. She was breaking my heart. I was up with her until 2 in the morning because she would not stop crying; Uncle Nate stepped in again and eventually got her to sleep. That was the hardest thing I had to do in my life. Rayleigh loved her grandma more than anything in this world. It crushed her little heart.

Blog entry from Ashley April 11th, 2014-

"I did the hardest thing I have ever had to do in my life. I sat next to my mommy, held her hand, kissed her forehead, told her how much I loved her and then told her it was okay to go. Even though she didn't respond I know she heard me. I told her not to worry about us. We will all be fine, which is a big fat lie. I have dreaded this moment and I never thought it would come so soon. I am tired of seeing her suffer. She needs to go in peace knowing that we will all be okay I love you mom!"

I never imagined at twenty eight years old I would be sitting next to my mother in a hospital bed telling her it is okay to die. As much as I did not want to tell her I knew I had to. I have seen so many patients hold on and suffer just for the simple fact that one family member did not come to see them or tell them it was okay to pass on, that everything would be okay. I was not going to let my mom lay there and suffer any longer because even in her condition she was still worried about everyone else but herself. She then sat up out of a dead sleep.

"Rayleigh!" Mom said

"What about her?" I asked

"She is outside by herself and you need to go get her."

"No she isn't mom she is in the other room with dad."

"No she is outside I heard her. Go get her." Mom snapped.

So I yelled for Ray to come into the living room and showed mom that she was inside and okay. The children that she heard were the kids from next door. Mom could barely sit up, speak or keep her eyes open at this point and she was still worried about where the kids were. God love my mother!

Blog entry from Nathan April 11th, 2014-

"Sitting here next to one of the strongest women I have ever known, holding her hand and just thinking about everything that she has taught me. She took on children that she did not birth. She never thought of me as a step son, she always introduced as, ""This is my son Nate."" I was never less than her own children and I love you for that, you have a huge part of my heart Tina and you always will, you are my angel, we watch over you and soon you will watch over us! I love you!"

This week was the week from hell; Tina played opossum like no other. Just when we thought she was about to go any minute, something would change. Mom would wake up, talking and laughing like before, and then crash again. Her pain become out of control again, the nurse got an order from the doctor allowing me to judge what dose of morphine I gave to mom so I would not have to keep calling them every other day to change it. Since mom was now unable to swallow her pills the nurse took her off of everything except the liquid morphine. My mother was okay with this until one day when Jamie came over and made the comment that mom did not need all of the pain medicine and she needed to be taking her pills again. When it was time to give mom her pain medicine she would not take it.

"What is wrong?" I asked

"I don't want that shit you are trying to kill me." Mom said hatefully.

"What are you talking about mom?"

"Jamie said that I don't need to be taking all of this pain medicine that you are just trying to drug me." This is not what Jamie said to her, he did however say the medicine was making mom too drugged and he didn't think she needed as much of it.

"Well mother no offense to Jamie but I have been in the medical field longer than he has been able to work. Your doctor and nurse both think that you need this. If I was going to kill you I would have done it by now, I have enough medicine in there right now to kill the whole entire family and probably some of our neighbors.'

"I don't care I am not taking them.' She snapped.

"Fine!' I yelled "Just lay there in pain then it is your choice and I am not fighting with you anymore!"

How could my mom think that I would ever hurt her? I was so hurt by what she said to me, and I was so damn pissed off at him. I called Jamie and told him that he needed to get his ass out here and talk to her. Mom's best friend Lorie came over that night and gave mom a stern talking to, after seeing the massive rug burn she gave herself from moving around in the bed due to being in so much pain. Lorie talked mom into taking a half of a dose of the morphine, it was something but not enough. When I tried to give mom another dose of the morphine later she slapped it out of my hand. I was at my wits end! Jamie came out the next night to take care of her so I could get a break because at this point I was ready to put a pillow over my mother's head as bad as that sounds, I could not do it anymore. I just wanted to curl up in a ball and cry. Jamie had a rude awakening and got a true taste of what being a care giver is all about. Mom was so uncomfortable and in so much pain that Jamie had to reposition her every five minutes. Just the few hours I had been asleep mom had completely wore him out.

"Dude, I have no idea how you have been doing this, mom is killing me." Jamie said.

"I told you, you thought that I was joking. Nothing you do works except her pain medicine that she refuses to take now." I said.

"You are right she needs it. I am seriously going to tie her to this bed if she does not sit still."

"Well then you need to tell her that you were wrong and to take her pain medicine."

Jamie finally talked mom into taking her pain medicine, I was not taking any chances I gave it to her right away. I called the nurse and let her know that mom was being aggressive. The nurse received orders from the doctor to give mom Haldol and Klonopin, my instructions were to give the Haldol then four hours later give the Klonopin. I was to crush them up and mix them in with the morphine. She also wanted me to up mom's dose from 20 milligrams every four hours to 40 milligrams every four hours. My Aunt Tammy came over later that afternoon and spent the night with mom so dad and I could both get some sleep. I prefilled enough syringes with medicine to get my aunt through the night so that she did not have to mess with it. Aunt Tammy got mom to do more than any of us had. I think maybe we made mom mad. That next morning before my aunt had to leave we gave mom a bath, it took everything we both had in us to move mom around to get her clean. The nurse had talked mom into a catheter a few days prior since Tina's kidneys were starting to fail drastically, as we were moving the catheter around to position mom I noticed her urine looked almost brown. I knew it would not be too much longer for her. At this point I knew it was going to be almost impossible for me to handle mom physically on my own. Her left side was way too weak.

Jamie and Nikki came out to visit with mom because we thought that we were about to lose her. Tina's breathing was very labored and shallow. Once mom heard Nikki's voice her eyes shot wide open and she started to wiggle and squirm in the bed.

"What is wrong mom?" I asked

"To leave" She mumbled.

"Who is leaving? You?" I said.

"Nikki" Said mom.

"Nikki isn't leaving mom don't worry."

"No" Mom said while shaking her head. "To leave."

"Do you want her to leave?" I asked.

"Yes" Tina muttered.

"Why do you want Nikki to leave mom?"

"The baby will get hurt, with me dying, the stress"

"Oh, you think that her seeing you like this is too much stress on her and the baby and you want her to go home?" I asked.

"Yes" mom said.

I went and told Jamie and Nikki what mom said. We were all laughing and crying at the same time. Tina was more worried about everyone else as always.

Blog entry from Nikki April 13th, 2014-

"Leave it to Tina to still be thinking of others even in her last days. She wanted me to go home today because she said her passing is too much stress on me and the baby. She is such a beautiful person inside and out, and I am so glad I got to know her! <3"

Blog entry from Amanda April 13th, 2014-

"Thanks to Becky and Joe I had the privilege of spending another weekend with my precious mother in law. I know soon she will no longer be with us here on earth but even now we get to have some great memories still being made to carry forever. This is very hard on everyone who loves her and there are many who love her! Bryon, Tina loves you so much, cherish the moments left even if it is just holding her hand and try to let tomorrow wait until tomorrow. Ashley, you are doing so much more for your mom than she can ever say, you are strong and you can do this. Jamie, hug your mom and hold her and let her know you will be okay, she loves you so much. Damon you have grown so much through all this, learn from it and make your mom proud, she worries about you. Nate you have such a gentle heart for Tina and she knows how much you love her."

Everyone went back home later that afternoon; I jumped back into taking care of mom. Amanda gave mom a bell to ring if she needed anything and we were not in the room. I speak for both dad and myself when I say Amanda should have had that bell shoved up her ass. I don't know how many times we threatened her about it. My mom was scared to be left alone at all; I was unable to leave the room for five minutes to use the bathroom. All I heard the whole time was mom trying to yell and the bell ringing like crazy. I knew after about thirty minutes of mom taking her morphine that she would sleep anywhere from thirty minutes to an hour. This was crunch time for me. I showered, went to the bathroom and did what little cleaning I could before she woke up. If I left mom's line of sight her anxiety would fly through the roof. The anxiety got to the point that mom was not even sleeping, even after she took the morphine. Tina was trying to fight off her medicine, was crawling out of bed and ripping the pillows out from underneath of her. I was afraid that mom would pull out her catheter or fall out of the bed. I called the nurse and explained to her what was going on and nothing I did was helping mom. She instructed me to start giving mom the morphine every single hour but to continue with the Haldol and Klonopin as before. I thought I was exhausted before, I had no idea what exhausted was until we started giving her medicine everyone hour. Tina's nurse brought me over a few more syringes so I could prefill more at a time now, even then it did not help the fact I had to be awake every single hour on the hour to give mom medicine. At one point I had been awake for sixty six hours. I was a walking zombie. The moment I thought mom was asleep and I tried to rest a bit before her next dose she would wake up and either ring the bell or start yelling for me. I prefilled 8 hours worth of syringes for dad and on his night off he stayed up with mom so I could get some sleep. I was in tears, falling asleep sitting up. I was so tired. I physically and mentally could not do it anymore.

Wednesday April 16th, 2014- Mom went unresponsive on us tonight; I called everyone because I thought that she only had a few short hours with us. Jamie got in his car and drove way over the speed limit to make it to the house to be with mom. Tina was very comfortable, I had been doing fairly well keeping on top of her medicine so she was not in pain. The nurse stopped by to check in on mom and her vital signs had dropped. There was a strong pulse but the blood pressure was almost undetectable. Mom's nurse and I both agreed only a few hours left. I did not want Rayleigh at the house and made arrangements with her father to come get her. They were unable to make it until Saturday; I knew we didn't have until Saturday. I called my best friend Kristina and asked her if she would be able to keep Rayleigh for the night, that we were not expecting mom to make it. Krissy came shortly after and picked up Ray, I don't know what I would have done without her. Not too long after mom bounced back but not much. I kept on top of her medicine as scheduled, mom slept very well that night. There was no anxiety at all. I sat next to her and held her hand.

"Momma why are you holding on? It is time for you to let go." I said.

My mom had barely spoken in days. She opened her eyes wider than I had seen them in days and she squeezed my hand.

"I am not and it will be time when it is time."

Mom closed her eyes and fell back asleep. I started crying, I did not think I would hear her voice again. Tina opened her eyes again.

"Don't cry, smile." She whispered

"I can't smile mom, there is nothing for me to smile about."

She then took her right hand reached across her body and hooked her finger into my mouth, pulling my cheek upwards.

"Damnit, I said smile."

I started crying and laughing at the same time.

"Damn you mom." I laughed "Even on your death bed you can still make everything okay."

"Even when I am gone I will."

That was the last time I heard my mother's voice. A conversation I will never forget and hold dear to my heart. My mother's last words to me tell you exactly what type of person she was. "Even when I am gone I will." She cared so much about her family. I wish I had known this would be the last time I talked to her. I would have made it a little longer and more meaningful. Thinking about it now I honestly do not know how much more meaningful it could have been. Her last words said it all.

At some point during the day mom had suffered from another stroke that took out her entire right side. She was unable to move on her own or speak at all.

Thursday April 17th, 2014- Today was mom's baby sister's birthday. I know my Aunt Missy did not enjoy this day at all. Most of her day was spent at the house with her sister. Several times we told mom please not today, please not today. I did not want my aunt's birthday to be the day she lost her sister, nobody wants that. The day was pretty routine for the most part. Later on that night Jamie and I were repositioning mom. I looked down at her legs, then her chest and arms.

"What are you doing?" Jamie asked.

"I am looking to see if she is mottling yet."

"What in the hell is that?" He asked.

"It is where the blood builds up in the vessels because it is not being pumped through the body properly, her skin will turn a purplish red color and will almost look like little circles touching each other."

"That is weird, what does it mean." He asked.

"Usually it is a sign they are close to death, the heart isn't pumping the blood like it should. People live with mottled skin all the time though."

"Is she mottled?" He asked

"No not yet." I said.

I went outside to call my boyfriend Lee; I had been out there maybe 10-15 minutes when Jamie came flying out of the front door.

"You need to get in here now Ashley mom's entire body just turned purple."

"Lee I have to let you go I will call you back." I said.

"No" He said "I heard him and I am on my way to your house, I will see you in a bit."

I don't think I even told Lee good-bye or that I loved him I just hung up the phone. I walked in and saw from the door that my mom's face was mottled.

"Holy shit Jamie! When did this happen?" Her whole entire body had mottled in less than fifteen minutes. I have never in my ten years of being a nursing assistant seen someone's whole body mottle that quickly.

"It was literally right before my eyes, her whole body; it was the craziest thing I had ever seen."

I called Nathan to let him know that we did not think that mom was going to make it through the night. He was in tears and said he was coming down right away. I talked him out of it because it was a four hours drive and I knew we didn't have four hours, not to mention the fact he had just got home from being on the road, He drives a semi and just finished up a trip to Memphis. He was exhausted and I did not want him to drive that far, that late on no sleep. I promised to keep him updated on how she was doing.

Jamie and I repositioned mom to make her more comfortable and I noticed that her bed was soaked. The catheter was leaking badly. I called the on call hospice nurse and explained to her what had gone on in the past thirty minutes or so. The nurse said that she would be on her way shortly. As we went to finish repositioning I noticed as we moved her she would turn grey and stop breathing.

"Stop!" I yelled at Jamie.

"What?" He said

"Don't touch her again; wait until the nurse gets here. I am warning you right now mom is not going to make it through this."

"How do you know?" He asked.

"Watch" I said as I lowered the head of her bed a little. His eyes got huge.

"Oh my god! Raise her back up hurry Ashley!" He screamed.

Friday April 18th, 2014- It took the nurse about an hour to arrive at the house. By this time it was passed midnight and onto a new day. She came in checked mom vitals, which she was unable to read, mom was only taking about five to six breaths a minute at this point.

"I am going to lay her head back so that I can remove your mom's catheter." The nurse said. As she started to lay mom's head backwards I noticed that mom completely stopped breathing.

"Stop!" I yelled "Don't touch her!"

"Why?" Asked the nurse.

"She is not going to make it through this and I don't want my mother to pass away while someone is yanking a catheter out of her vagina. Let her be!"

Jamie started to cry as mom slowly turned from pink to grey and her body went limp and cold. We all stood around in silence, holding her hands. At 12:25 am on April 18th, 2014 my mother Tina took her last breath here on this earth. She had gotten her wish, to pass away at home surrounded by friends and family.

Jamie looked over at me in tears.

"Is she?" He asked.

"Yea bud, she is gone." I said.

My dad and Lee had stepped outside on the porch while Jamie and I were helping the nurse with mom. I walked outside, dad looked over at me and all I could do was shake my head up and down. He knew she was gone. The nurse called it in and the official time of death was 12:41am. My mom had waited until Aunt Missy's birthday was over. Jamie, Dad, Aunt Missy, Lee, Nikki, Jamie's best friend Kevin and I all stood around mom's body as Kevin fought through the tears to say one last prayer for her. Dad called his best friend T.C. who lived just down the street; he came over to be with dad. Dad and I both talked to Nathan and let him know she had passed away. He completely lost it, we could barely understand him though the crying. He kept saying he should have been here with her. Dad and I both told him it was okay, that mom understood why he was not here. We would have rather him stayed at home safe and in one piece then drive down here like a bad out of hell and leave us with two funerals. I then called my Aunt Tammy and mom's friend Carla to let them know she was no longer with us. I could not stand to hear them cry but I knew it had to be done. About an hour later the funeral home came to get mom's body. I stood in the door as they loaded her from the bed to the stretcher. It felt as if I was there for hours. I just stood there numb staring off into space. This was it, she was gone. It didn't seem real until I looked over and the funeral home directors were walking out of the front door with my mom's body covered in a blanket. Dad came up next to me and put his arm on my shoulder.

"It will be okay." He said crying.

"It doesn't seem real." I said

"I know" dad said he then kissed my forehead. "I just want you to know how proud I am of you, I could not have done this without your help and I know your mom is proud of you."

I ran out the door to Lee who was standing on the front porch, I grabbed him tightly and just cried. I was so glad he was there. Dad came walking around the side of the house a few minutes later, whiter than a ghost.

"What is wrong with you?" I asked

"That frog your mom bought last summer that would not light up, it is lit up brighter than hell."

"You are messing with me." I said

"I am not, go look."

Lee and I walked around back and sure enough it was lit up and extremely bright. That morning I received a message from a family friend of ours named Pam. Her husband was killed when I was around junior high age in a biking accident. Ever since J.T. had passed away Pam and her family had these odd run ins with ladybugs. When she saw the frog statue was lit up she bought me a frog key chain to hang from my window in my car. I wanted to cry when she handed it to me. She said it reminded her of her ladybugs.

Blog entry from Ashley April 18th, 2014-

"My mom is with us. She bought this frog last summer and it has not worked since she got it. Dad did everything to make this frog light up. Early this morning after mom passed, dad walked around back to a lit up frog! We got your message mommy!!!"

Later that night Dad, Jamie, Nathan, Kevin and I all went to Uncle Monkey's a restaurant in town for dinner; they did not let us pay for our meals. It was very nice of them do that for us. We then headed to Bunker's for drinks which we all needed at this point. Word had spread fast about mom's passing and we were flooded with visits, calls and text messages. It was just an overwhelming day to say the least. We all had several people come up to us and offer their condolences, tell us stories about their family members and how to cope. I am glad I live in such a small community because my family had so much support during this time, we needed it!

Blog entry from Ashley April 19th, 2014-

"Hey mom, the cubs won today! Thanks!"

My mom hated the Chicago Cubs, when I heard they had won, I knew it was her doing. It made me smile.

Blog entry from Nathan April19th, 2014-

"Yesterday was a horrible day, but also a blessing! Heaven received an angel Tina, a great loving caring honest and beautiful woman. My father Bryon, my sister Ashley and my brother Jamie, it was tough to be in the house, difficult to not wake up to a woman that asked ""Would you guys like some breakfast?"" or ""Hey wake your ass up, you are not sleeping all day long."" Just always making sure we were all okay. The difficulty will still continue as we prepare to lay her to rest in the days to come, but with each other we can get through this together, we have gotten through this thus far and if we can do this, we can get through anything. This was the hardest thing we have ever had to deal with but she is in a better place with no pain, no discomfort and no worries. She would be the first person to tell us she is fine, not to cry and to be honest she is probably still worried about us. But we will get through this heartache, this pain of a beautiful person inside and out taken away from us to soon. We had some good laughs and good talks about memories of Tina last night with great friends that have been so supportive to my family. Bringing us over food, flowers or just stopping by to check on us, this is truly a great community. We got dad out of the house last night for some dinner and to just take some time to breath. Thank you to Uncle Monkey's for dinner! Thank you to this community and thank you to great friends. It has really made our time with Tina and now our time without so much easier! I love you dad, Ashley and Jamie, we will always have our memories! R.I.P. Tina June 28th, 1964-April 18th, 2014. We love you and will always miss you!"

Blog entry from Ashley April 19th, 2014-

"I have so many people to thank, first off my dad Bryon for being so strong when life was kicking you in the ass. To my brothers Jamie, Nathan and Damon for stepping up and pulling together when we should have all fallen apart. We are all so much closer now and I love you. To my boyfriend Lee for dealing with my emotions and standing by my side as I watched my mom slip away. You are the most amazing man I have ever met and I could not have done this without you! I love you! My sister in law Amanda, Debbie M., My Aunt Jenny and my Aunt Tammy for helping take some of the load off of our shoulders by sitting with mom and all of those who offered. To Alyson I don't even remember why we were mad at each other honestly; I am glad you came up and hugged me and said how stupid we were both being. We were so close for a while and I have missed you terribly it was a huge relief and helped a lot. I love you to death. Leslie…. Leslie Leslie Leslie god I hated your ass growing up, but yet you were in a sense my idol. I wanted to be as good as you in volleyball and you pushed to make me a better player even though you weren't aware of it. We are much older now and I am over all of this mean high school stuff. You coming up to me last night, hugging me and telling me the story of your mom showed me you are not the mean cold hearted person I thought that you were and for that I am sorry I have been such a rude bitch to you every time I have seen you. It meant so much to me; my own family has not called to check up on me, so thank you for that! You are alright in my book! Adam I was so depressed last night and our talk of the past and all of the stupid shit we did put a smile on my face; I have not smiled in a long time. To everyone who has brought food, stopped by and given donations, thank you all so much for making this life shattering event so much easier to make peace with! I have reconnected with people I never imagined I'd ever speak to again. So in this tragic loss I have gained a lot!! I love you all for your support!!"

Saturday April 26th, 2014- Today was mom's memorial service. Mom was cremated and dad got a plain wooden urn to put her ashes in. When the kids arrived the morning of the service they all took a side of the urn and decorated it with mom's left over stickers from her scrap booking supplies. My sister-in-law Amanda made everyone white ribbon pins to wear in mom's honor. Everyone gathered up their speeches and headed to the church. It was packed full by the time my family arrived and people were still coming in. There was no room in there to sit or stand. Reverend Melissa came to the podium, welcomed everyone and started off with mom's obituary.

"Tina Marie Honea of Illiopolis IL passed away peacefully in her home on April 18th, 2014 at 12:41 am. Tina was the daughter of Merle Harp of Springfield IL, Daughter-in-law of Juanita Conyers of Taylorville IL. She is survived by her husband Bryon Honea of Illiopolis, children, Rocky the dog (her favorite child), Nathan (Amanda) Honea of Harvard IL, Ashley Honea of Illiopolis IL, James Honea of Decatur IL, Damon Honea of Illiopolis IL, Bryon (Ashley) Honea of Peoria IL, Jason (Jessica) Honea of Woodstock IL, Daniel (Meghan) Honea of Wonderlake IL. Her 12 grandbabies, Brianna, Bradley, Destiny, Dylan, Rayleigh, Jaycee, Noah, Nolan, Lexie, Bryce, Krue, and Rylan. Sisters Tammy (Jeff) Cooper of New Holland IL, Melissa Harp of Springfield IL. Sister-in-law Jennifer (Jim) Graham of Taylorville IL. Tina was an avid scrap booker and loved to garden. She was a children's librarian for years, later going to Riverton Elementary as a para educator. Tina loved being around children and was loved by all she crossed paths with. A memorial service for Tina will be held at the Illiopolis Christian Church on

April 26th, at 2:00pm and burial for Tina will be held at a later date for close family and friends."

        Melissa read a few prayers and then was going to play an Ozzy Ozborne song by dad's request. Mom hated Ozzy with a passion. The P.A. system in the church stopped working at that moment. The CD would play but there was no sound. Well played mom! We all laughed, mom always told him she did not want that crap played at her funeral, and apparently she meant it! One of mom's friends Kathy got up to the podium and read a book for the kids, to help them better understand mom's body being gone but her spirit still being with us. Kathy is great with kids; she was the perfect person to help them all understand. Nathan and I took turns reading speeches the family had written. Nathan wrote:

        "Tina Marie Honea, Born June 28th 1964, passed on April 18th 2014. She married my father on October 19th 1985. Some of you may not know this but Tina did not have any children when her and my dad married. My dad had 4 sons Bryon, Jason, Myself and Daniel. She took us in as if we were her own children. Over the last few weeks with everything that has been going on with Tina whether it be Facebook messages, the car show we had in Mechanicsburg or the get together we had at the mini mall in Illiopolis, a lot of people have sent me messages or come up to me and said "I never knew you weren't Tina's real son". She never introduced us as her step children, it was always," These are my sons" I felt sorry for you if you ever said, "Oh this is your step son right?" because she would be the first one to tell you, "These are my sons." Tina was a wonderful person and a wonderful mother to all of her children and to friends of ours. She never put herself first even through all of this; she always put everyone else first making sure that they were ok. Even in her final days she would still say, "Are you doing ok, how are the grandbabies and don't you dare cry" She was the toughest woman I have ever met, she fought this monster longer than a lot of people ever could. Tina Loved the Dallas Cowboys and the St. Louis Cardinals, though I'm not sure why. She loved to scrapbook, take pictures with her camera, and hang out with family, especially her grandbabies. To my sister Ashley and my brothers Jamie and Damon, you guys are rocks, with countless hours of no sleep and being by her side day in and day out. To make sure that she had everything that she needed to be comfortable. To Amanda, a woman that never left Tina's side whether it be here or when she came and stayed at our house up north. I watched you do everything for the woman and I thank you from the bottom of my heart. She truly appreciated it and always asked where you were when I came down here by myself. To this community, I cannot begin to express the appreciation, love and comfort that we have felt from you. With the kid kind loving words, cards and all the food that has been sent to the house my dad almost needed to get another fridge. This is a great community with tons of friends, we are truly grateful for all that you have done for us. And to my father, you are the strongest man I have ever and will ever know, to watch you or talk to you every day, when we needed to talk, vent or just cry we were there for each other, we all were. Our life has forever been changed but we keep the memories with us, we keep her close to our heart and we look to the sky to see her. She would not want us to cry, she would want us to be sad, Tina's biggest concern was that she didn't know if we were going to be ok after she had passed. I told her, like I have always told her; we are Honeas we can get through anything. Though it is going to be tough, she would want us to carry on, carry on her memories and with the friends and family that we

have I think we can do just that. I love you Tina Marie Honea, we really have the best guardian angel!!"

It was hard to get up there and see everyone crying. Our speeches were filled with jokes and memories of the good times. We did not want to make them sad but rather happy to brighten the mood as much as possible.

After the service the family escorted everyone to the dining hall for a dinner that the wonderful ladies of the church put on for us. Dinner was delicious! Afterwards dad and I walked back in to look at all of moms flowers everyone sent. A few of them were beautiful and had nice messages.

"To the Honea family, from your friends at the Illiopolis Fast Stop. Karen, Jodi, Cassy, Jennifer, Nick, Denise and Alyssa."

"With deepest sympathy. Patty, Krystal and Alyvia."

"To the woman who always treated me as her own. We will love and miss you. Jason, Jessica, Nolan and Lexie Honea"

There were probably ten bouquets of flowers total; my Aunt Jenny took most of them home with her. She has a friend who makes beads from the flowers. We all have necklaces, bracelets and key chains made from the flowers at mom's service. They have to be one of the neatest things I have ever seen.

Blog entry from Ashley May 9th, 2014-

"It has been three weeks, yet it feels like an eternity. It is just not the same with you not around. I see your pictures and try to pretend you are still here, when I open my eyes you will be sitting across from me. I miss you more than words can explain! I love you momma! Fly high!"

Once mom's services were over, dad had to change the house around in order for him to be able to stay there. One night him and I were painting and had went outside to take a break. As we are standing on the porch we hear the loudest frog we have ever heard in our lives. He and I quietly tip toe back to the pool and dad shines his light into the bottom and it is filled with frogs. I have never seen a frog in the pool in all of the years my parents have had one up and now it is filled with them. Dad just stood there shaking his head. He knew it was mom. Things from then on got really weird, thankfully Lee and T.C. were around to see them or no one would have believed us. One night we had a paint scraper and a stack of papers go flying across the room and no one was standing by them. Stuff was falling off the walls and counters. If anyone would take pictures in the house it would have a bright white streak through it or looked foggy. None of these things ever happened until mom passed away. We now hear what sounds like footsteps especially at night. Rocky will sit in front of the chair where mom used to sit and bark and growl. He never barks or growls.

Blog entry from Jamie May 11th, 2014-

"For those of you who think it is just another day and don't spend time with your mother. There are some of us who can't spend this day with ours and would do anything to spend it with them. So while you have the chance still make the days like today special! I love you and miss you terribly mom!"

This was a tough day. None of us knew what to do, it had always been about my mom. We all hopped into the car and went to my grandma's house. We had lunch and spent the day laughing and joking. It was a great day but there was a huge piece missing, mom. Later that night I was helping my dad clean some of mom's belongs out of the house and I came across a hand written journal that mom started when she found out she had cancer. I wish I had known about this sooner and wish she would have written in it more than she did, especially towards the end since none of us really knew what was going on in her head.

It was titled My Journey

"June 12th, 2012 was the beginning of my journey. After several months of having a very agonizing pain in my left shoulder, I was finally getting some answers at the hospital after 3 trips to the E.R. with no real answers. Bryon took me to the E.R. on 6/13/12 the pain was so bad nothing was working. After 3 trips an x-ray was done to show a mass in my left lung. Within 30 minutes I was off to have a CT scan. The CT scan confirmed the 6 to7 centimeter mass. I was put into isolation and told I would be transported to Springfield. Later that afternoon on 6/13/12 I was transported to Springfield where I again was put into isolation. They weren't sure what the mass was, but they were thinking 1 of 3 things 1. T.B. 2.Leptospirosis 3. Lung cancer."

"6-14-12 more blood work done and tests taken. No answers yet. Bronchial biopsy done."

"6-15-12 Doctors came into my room this afternoon with a diagnosis of lung cancer. They sounded very grim. I am a fighter so let the battle begin. I have 9 beautiful reasons to fight for my life. My family are all here with and for me. This is the important thing."

"6-16-12 came home from the hospital. A lot of changes lie ahead for me. With the love of God and my family I can win this battle."

"6-18-12 at the doctors the game plan is to remove the tumor from my left lung on 7-24-12 Diagnosis stage 3A."

"6-19-12 bathroom is being replaced this weekend. I am so excited!"

"6-28-12 today is my 48th birthday and my monkey is here spending a few days with maw maw and paw paw. Tonight Belle, Dick, Tammy, Bryon, Jamie, Monkey and I are going to Texas Roadhouse for my birthday steak dinner. What a wonderful evening it was at Texas Roadhouse with the people that I love. My steak was awesome; I even had a raspberry margarita YUM! Tammy bought me some cute wall hangers and Belle and Dick paid for everyone's dinner. I am so blessed to have these people in my life."

"7-3-12 Nate came to get me for a few days so I can spend time with my babies. Off to Harvard I go for a week."

"7-9-12 back home, brought Brianna, Bradley and Destiny home with me for the week. I love having my babies around."

That was the last entry she wrote in the journal. It was not much but pulling this out of the box next to her chair that she had it hidden in made me smile and cry. It was almost like having a piece of mom right there with me. I felt like I got to have one more moment with her. I called dad and all of the boys and read it to them over the phone. It was a bittersweet moment.

Blog entry from Ashley June 21st, 2014-

"I was walking through the hallway at work tonight and I heard a Reba song on one of my resident's televisions, I got a little teary eyed because of course it automatically makes me think of mom. As I am walking outside this frog jumps onto the window seal right next to the door! Thanks mom!"

We have had several run ins with frogs since mom's passing. They all happen to be in times of sadness or stress. I was a huge skeptic about people coming to you in the form of animals, bugs or inanimate objects, I am a believer now all of the way. There have been too many occurrences not to be a believer. My mom loved frogs, it makes perfect sense.

Blog entry from Nathan June 28th, 2014-

"You were taken away from us too soon! Today would have been only your 50th birthday; you should have had so many more years left with us. I love you Tina. I think about you every day and miss you terribly; happy birthday and I love you with all of my heart!!"

Blog entry from Ashley June 28th, 2014-

"Happy birthday to the best lady in the world, I hope you are having one hell of a party up there! Love you momma, Fly high!"

Today mom would have been 50. It was one of her last wishes, to make it to her 50th birthday, which she fell just shy of. Mom had so many plans and trips she wanted to take once she reached her 50th, it was almost as if she were starting her bucket list if you will. I am saddened that mom never got to do the things in life she wanted. I wish there were a way I could have made them all happen for her. With that being said, despite everything she wanted to do, my mom had a life full of happiness and cheer. She had the chance to meet many famous people, go to concerts and places she had always wanted to visit. Even though her list was not 100 percent complete she was happy and fulfilled when she went.

Blog entry from Damon July 24th, 2014-

"Dear mom, I have really needed you there past few months. I have so much going on and there is no one around to talk to. I wake up every single day just hoping it is the end of the horrible nightmare and that I can just call and get everything out, I can't believe you are gone. I miss you and love you so so much!"

I think out us all Damon had the hardest time with mom's passing, he was not there with her when she passed due to some personal issues of his own he was dealing with. I know he beats himself up every day for not being there by her side. I am glad he was not. He was the baby and got away with murder around my mom. Those two fought more than any of us but they were the closest. I am glad he does not have the memory of my mom taking her last breath in his head. I think that would have devastated him to a point there would be no coming back.

It has been four months since we lost my mother. Not one day goes by that I do not wish she were here with me. She was my best friend, I turned to her for everything and she always had an answer. It may not have been the answer that I was looking for but there was one offered to me, and it was always just what I needed to hear. Things will never be the same without her around. We have all moved on and are healing but we have not forgotten nor will we ever. We have so many things to be grateful for, our children, friends and family. Although mom is not physically here I know she is with us. I see frogs all the time and I can't help but smile. I know it is her way of saying hello.

Cancer is something that we all have to deal with and it is never easy. You are going to be in for one hell of a ride whether you are the patient or the family; it is not easy no matter what position you are in. We have to stand strong and fight through these tough times if we are going to make it. I hope that each of you reading this that are or will have to deal with this nasty monster take one thing from this story and that is never ever give up hope, never quit, and never quit caring. You are strong, you can do this and you will make it in the end if your loved one does lose the fighting battle. Always remember one thing, how will they fly high if we don't carry on their memories?